Handbook of Evidence-Based Stereotactic Radiosurgery and Stereotactic Body Radiotherapy

W0112655

Rajni A. Sethi • Igor J. Barani
David A. Larson • Mack Roach III
Editors

Handbook of Evidence-Based Stereotactic Radiosurgery and Stereotactic Body Radiotherapy

Second Edition

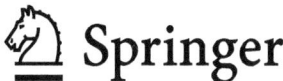 Springer

Editors

Rajni A. Sethi
Department of Radiation
Oncology
Kaiser Permanente
Dublin, CA, USA

Igor J. Barani
Department of Radiation
Oncology
Barrow Neurological Institute
Phoenix, AZ, USA

David A. Larson
San Francisco, CA, USA

Mack Roach III
Department of Radiation
Oncology and Urology
University of California, San
Francisco
San Francisco, CA, USA

ISBN 978-3-031-33155-8   ISBN 978-3-031-33156-5   (eBook)
https://doi.org/10.1007/978-3-031-33156-5

This Springer imprint is published by the registered company Springer
Nature Switzerland AG
The registered company address is: Gewerbestrasse 11, 6330 Cham, Switzerland

In Memoriam: Dr. David Andrew Larson, PhD, MD

This book is a heartfelt dedication to the memory of Dr. David Andrew Larson, a distinguished and accomplished individual whose profound contributions to the fields of physics and radiation oncology continue to resonate within the medical community.

Born in Astoria, Oregon, in 1940, Dave's insatiable thirst for knowledge manifested early in his life. His intellectual journey began at UC Berkeley, where he majored in physics and earned the esteemed title of top physics student in his class.

Continuing his pursuit of academic excellence, Dave furthered his studies in astrophysics at Columbia University. He later obtained a master's degree in particle physics and a Ph.D. in high energy physics from the University of Chicago. His doctoral research was remarkable, yielding valuable insights and constraints on theoretical models for the distri-

bution of pions detected in the Earth's atmosphere from outer space particles.

After seven productive years at Cornell and Harvard, where he engaged in experimental elementary particle physics research, Dave's unwavering dedication led him to embark on a transformative career change. He entered an accelerated medical school program at the University of Miami School of Medicine, completing his medical degree in just two years.

Dave's medical career brought him to the Joint Center for Radiation Therapy at Harvard and later, to the University of California, San Francisco (UCSF), where he honed his expertise in radiation oncology. He spent 34 distinguished years at UCSF, spearheading the treatment of brain tumors and pioneering groundbreaking radiosurgery programs, where he saved the lives of countless patients and set new standards in the field.

Dave's commitment to medical advancements extended beyond his clinical practice. He served as President of the American Society for Therapeutic Radiation Oncology (ASTRO) and the International Radiosurgery Society, leaving a lasting impact on the global oncology community.

Dave was a devoted family man. As a father to Whitney, Colin, and Jeremy, he infused his children's lives with love, support, and endless adventures. Dave's profound impact on their growth and development was immeasurable, as he instilled in them values of integrity, kindness, and humility.

As we bid farewell to this exceptional individual, let us remember and honor Dr. David Andrew Larson for his trailblazing contributions to physics and medicine, and for the profound love and kindness he bestowed upon his family and friends. This dedication serves as a testament to the legacy he leaves behind and a reminder of the transformative power of a life lived with purpose and compassion.

Preface to the Second Edition

The first edition of the *Handbook of Evidence-Based Stereotactic Radiosurgery (SRS) and Stereotactic Body Radiotherapy (SBRT)* was published in 2016 with the intent to provide a concise go-to reference for practitioners of these techniques. In the years since the publication of the first edition, we have seen widespread adoption of SRS and SBRT in both academic and community-based centers worldwide. This has been fueled by multiple advancements. First, there is increased availability of highly sophisticated radiotherapy equipment and techniques including X-ray and MRI-based onboard imaging, in-room tumor-tracking systems, patient immobilization systems with real-time biofeedback, 4D image capture for treatment planning, beam gating, and complex treatment planning systems with enhanced algorithms and deformable image registration. Additionally, progress in clinical research has given clues as to the optimal scenarios in which these technologies can be most useful. As the practices of SRS and SBRT have continued to mature since their inception in the 1980s, their associated research compendium has grown beyond retrospective series and phase I/II clinical trials to include the recent publication of multiple randomized phase II and III clinical trials. Furthermore, our increasing interconnectedness and comfort using remote video-based secure applications, somewhat spurred by necessity during the Covid pandemic, have increased the incorporation of remote treatment management discussions and expert peer review. Finally, there are increasing educational opportunities for practitioners to learn how to safely employ these techniques, through annual symposia, fellowship opportunities, and publication of practical guidelines by our medical societies.

As a handbook, the nature of this publication is to be concise and easily referenced during a busy clinical day. As such, we have limited the amount of information included in each chapter. We encourage you to refer to original publications as listed in the reference section as well as clinical trial treatment protocols for more detailed information.

We continue to present the *Handbook of Stereotactic Radiosurgery and Stereotactic Body Radiotherapy* as a companion book to our institution's prior publication, *Handbook of Evidence-Based Radiotherapy*. As such, we have attempted not to replicate general information regarding anatomy, staging, workup, and follow-up for each disease site, which can be referenced in the latter. The current handbook focuses on specific uses of SRS and SBRT, with chapters organized by disease site. We include a description of treatment techniques and recommended imaging. We also address safety and quality assurance issues as well as toxicity and management issues specific to SRS and SBRT. We have also included an introductory chapter that elucidates the historical context of these techniques as well as a chapter explaining treatment delivery systems. Finally, in the appendix, we include a summary of normal tissue dose tolerances.

We initially developed this handbook to provide an easily accessible summary of typical practices and published results based on disease site. The current edition incorporates "lessons learned" as we continue to gain experience using these techniques. We present the results of recent publications, explain new technologies, and incorporate updated practice recommendations. Compared to the first edition, you will notice a stronger focus on clinical outcomes and practical recommendations. As with any concise reference or publication, there may be subtle details or ingredients left out that can critically impact the results. As such, we cannot and do not vouch for the safety of any of the treatment practices reported in this handbook. In all cases, clinical judgment is required, particularly in cases when dose-limiting structures are put at risk when adjacent to very high doses of radiation.

In many cases, the contents of this book reflect the treatment approach at the University of California at San Francisco, where early pioneers of SRS and SBRT gained expertise and over the years developed a rich and varied program to implement SRS and SBRT in many settings. This book is meant to summarize our own experience and that of our colleagues who have reported separately in peer-reviewed journals and at national and international meetings. Individual practitioners must use their own clinical judgment and knowledge to guide the use of SRS and SBRT in their own practice. Specifically, we caution against the use of these highly skilled techniques in institutions without prior training or expertise.

We want to sincerely thank the contributing authors for the excellent chapters they have produced. Thank you to our editors for their patience and encouragement and keeping us on track through this process. This handbook would not have been possible without their support and hours of hard work and dedication. We want to continue to acknowledge the pioneers in our field whose tenacity and ingenuity built the body of work that we are presenting here today, as we continue to move forward with the constant goal of improving outcomes for our patients. And finally, we want to thank our patients whose courage continues to inspire us every day.

Sincerely,

Dublin, CA   Rajni A. Sethi
Phoenix, AZ   Igor J. Barani
San Francisco, CA   Mack Roach III
San Francisco, CA   David A. Larson

Contents

1   **Introduction to Stereotactic Radiosurgery
    and Stereotactic Body Radiotherapy**   1
    David A. Larson

**Part I   Physics of Stereotactic Radiosurgery
           and Stereotactic Body Radiotherapy**

2   **Physics of Stereotactic Radiosurgery
    and Stereotactic Body Radiotherapy**   11
    Angélica Pérez-Andújar, Martina Descovich,
    and Cynthia Chuang

Part II   Clinical Applications

3   **Intracranial Tumors**   39
    Matthew S. Susko, Jessica Chew, Steve E. Braunstein,
    David A. Larson, and David R. Raleigh

4   **Spine**   89
    Jessica Chew, Matthew S. Susko, David R. Raleigh,
    Igor J. Barani, David A. Larson,
    and Steve E. Braunstein

5   **Head and Neck** 121
    Christina Phuong and Jason W. Chan

6   **Lung** 137
    Katelyn Hasse and Jason W. Chan

7   **Digestive System**.............................161
    Ting Martin Ma and Mekhail Anwar

8   **Genitourinary Sites** 209
    William C. Chen, Alexander R. Gottschalk,
    and Mack Roach III

9   **Gynecologic Sites** 233
    Matthew S. Susko, Rajni A. Sethi,
    Zachary A. Seymour, and I-Chow Joe Hsu

10 **Soft Tissue Sarcoma** 247
    Katherine S. Chen, Steve E. Braunstein,
    and Alexander R. Gottschalk

11 **Extracranial Oligometastases** 265
    William C. Chen and Steve E. Braunstein

Appendix A: Dose-Volume Criteria...................279

Index...291

Contributors

Mekhail Anwar Department of Radiation Oncology, University of California San Francisco, San Francisco, CA, USA

Igor J. Barani Department of Radiation Oncology, Barrow Neurological Institute, Phoenix, AZ, USA

Steve E. Braunstein Department of Radiation Oncology, University of California, San Francisco, San Francisco, CA, USA

Jason W. Chan Department of Radiation Oncology, University of California, San Francisco, San Francisco, CA, USA

Katherine S. Chen Department of Radiation Oncology, University of California, San Francisco, San Francisco, CA, USA

William C. Chen Department of Radiation Oncology, University of California, San Francisco, San Francisco, CA, USA

Jessica Chew Department of Radiation Oncology, University of California, San Francisco, San Francisco, CA, USA

Cynthia Chuang Radiation Oncology, Stanford University, Stanford, CA, USA

Martina Descovich Division of Physics, Department of Radiation Oncology, University of California, San Francisco, San Francisco, CA, USA

Alexander R. Gottschalk Department of Radiation Oncology, University of California, San Francisco, San Francisco, CA, USA

Katelyn Hasse Department of Radiation Oncology, University of California, San Francisco, San Francisco, CA, USA

I-Chow Joe Hsu Department of Radiation Oncology, University of California, San Francisco, San Francisco, CA, USA

David A. Larson (deceased), Departments of Radiation Oncology and Neurological Surgery, University of California, San Francisco, San Francisco, CA, USA

Ting Martin Ma Department of Radiation Oncology, University of California Los Angeles, Los Angeles, CA, USA

Angélica Pérez-Andújar Medical Physics, Memorial Sloan Kettering Cancer Center, West Harrison, NY, USA

Christina Phuong Department of Radiation Oncology, University of California, San Francisco, San Francisco, CA, USA

David R. Raleigh Departments of Radiation Oncology and Neurological Surgery, University of California, San Francisco, San Francisco, CA, USA

Mack Roach III Department of Radiation Oncology, University of California, San Francisco, San Francisco, CA, USA

Rajni A. Sethi Department of Radiation Oncology, Kaiser Permanente, Dublin, CA, USA

Zachary A. Seymour Department of Radiation Oncology, Beaumont Health, Sterling Heights, MI, USA

Matthew S. Susko Department of Radiation Oncology, University of California, San Francisco, San Francisco, CA, USA

Chapter 1
Introduction to Stereotactic Radiosurgery and Stereotactic Body Radiotherapy

David A. Larson

Stereotactic radiosurgery (SRS) and stereotactic body radiotherapy (SBRT) have a firmly established role in the management of malignant and benign conditions. They have dramatically altered the way clinicians think about target margins and fractionation, and therefore they rank among the most important historical advances in radiation oncology, including the development of megavoltage treatment machines, imaging-based treatment planning, and intensity-modulated radiation therapy. SRS and SBRT technologies were developed and implemented by dedicated clinicians and physicists (Benedict et al. 2008), and patient selection factors and clinical outcomes have become well established. As a result, SRS and SBRT are an important part of the knowledge base of practicing physicists and physicians and a critical part of the educational curriculum for radiation oncology residents.

_____

D. A. Larson (✉)
(deceased), Departments of Radiation Oncology and Neurological Surgery, University of California, San Francisco,
San Francisco, CA, USA
e-mail: DLarson@radonc.ucsf.edu

© The Author(s), under exclusive license to Springer Nature Switzerland AG 2023
R. A. Sethi et al. (eds.), *Handbook of Evidence-Based Stereotactic Radiosurgery and Stereotactic Body Radiotherapy*,
https://doi.org/10.1007/978-3-031-33156-5_1

Historical Foundations

During the 1950s, neuroanatomists and neurophysiologists developed techniques to produce small, highly localized, ablative CNS radio-lesions in animals using a variety of radiation sources, including implanted radon seeds, implanted isotopes such as Au^{198} and Co^{60}, betatron X-rays, and protons and deuterons. Swedish neurosurgeon Lars Leksell, a pioneer in the development of stereotaxy, recognized that small, accurately placed radio-lesions could be produced in humans. In 1951, he coined the term "radiosurgery" and is recognized as the father of radiosurgery (Leksell 1951). He performed focal single-fraction experiments in the brains of goats, cats, and rabbits using multiple cross-fired proton beams as he sought an optimum dose to produce discrete CNS lesions of dimension 3–7 mm. He found that a suitable maximum dose for the production of a discrete lesion within 1–2 weeks was 20 Gy in a single fraction. In the 1950s and 1960s, he pioneered X-ray and proton SRS for pain syndromes and movement disorders. In 1961, he used 3 mm cross-fired proton beams to perform thalamotomies for pain control. He invented the Gamma Knife and performed his first Gamma Knife procedure in 1967. In 1974, that first Gamma Knife was installed as an experimental tool at UCLA under the direction of neurosurgeon Bob Rand.

During the 1950s, in the USA, internist John Lawrence, often called the father of nuclear medicine, developed highly focal ablative radiation procedures with cyclotron-produced protons, deuterons, and helium ions at what is now called Lawrence Berkeley National Laboratory (where John's brother, Ernest, invented the cyclotron, for which he was awarded the Nobel Prize). He took great interest in pituitary disorders and performed multi-fraction dose/targeting studies in dogs, rats, and monkeys using bone landmarks to target and ablate the pituitary with multiple cross-fired non-Bragg peak beams. He initiated human studies in 1954, initially to suppress pituitary function in breast cancer patients and subsequently to treat acromegaly. He tried numerous fractionation schemes, eventually settling on 300 Gy in 6 fractions over 2 weeks to ablate the pituitary without damage to the surrounding tissue.

In 1961, Massachusetts General Hospital neurosurgeons William Sweet and Raymond Kjellberg initiated treatment of pituitary tumors and arteriovenous malformations with single-fraction Bragg-peak protons. Kjellberg searched the literature for examples of brain radionecrosis in humans, monkeys, and rats; plotted his findings as log of dose sufficient to produce necrosis versus log of beam diameter; and connected the data points with a steep straight line demonstrating the strong relationship between treatment volume and likelihood of necrosis. His plot indicated that 10 Gy was sufficient to produce necrosis for a 10 cm beam diameter and 4000 Gy was sufficient to produce necrosis for a 10 μm beam diameter (Kjelberg 1979). Many of his initial human SRS treatments involved doses considered just sufficient to cause radionecrosis, according to his necrosis plot.

In the 1980s, radiologist Jack Fabricant used Bragg peak heavy ions produced at the Berkeley cyclotron to treat hundreds of patients with arteriovenous malformations or pituitary disorders. At the same time, neurosurgeons in Europe, South America, and North America began developing SRS programs using modified linear accelerators or cobalt teletherapy units. One of the best known systems was the linac SRS system developed by the neurosurgeon Ken Winston and physicist Wendell Lutz in Boston, stimulated by the work of Leksell and designed to be capable of delivering very high, single-fraction photon radiation doses in the range of 100–150 Gy to small, precisely located, volumes (0.5–2 cm^3) within the brain (Lutz et al. 1984).

Development of SRS and SBRT

Although the above historical foundations involved focally ablative lesioning, SRS as it developed in the late 1980s involved less aggressive single-fraction maximum doses, in the range of 20–50 Gy for most indications and for treatment volumes up to about 15 cc, with higher maximum doses in the range of 100–150 Gy reserved for pain syndromes or movement disorders and for treatment volumes less than about 0.1 cc. Selection of the less aggressive doses was strongly influenced by radiation oncologists and neurosurgeons at the first North American SRS locations, including Boston (1/86, AVM), Montreal (12/86, AVM), Pittsburgh (8/87, acoustic neuroma), and San Francisco (3/88, AVM). Initial treatments at those facilities and others throughout the world were for benign rather than malignant indications, even though today the majority of SRS and nearly all SBRT procedures are for malignant processes. One of the first reported malignant indications receiving SRS was Sturm's 1987 report on brain metastasis (Sturm et al. 1987).

During the late 1980s and early 1990s, SRS grew rapidly. The first North American Radiosurgery conference was held in 1987 in Boston, organized by the neurosurgeon Ken Winston and radiation oncologist Jay Loeffler, attracting 100 registrants. ASTRO's first "refresher" course on radiosurgery, attended by about 400 members, was presented by the radiation oncologist David Larson at ASTRO's Annual Meeting in New Orleans in 1988. The yearly number of SRS patients in North America increased from about 600 in 1990 to about 12,000 in 2000, during which period the number of yearly publications on SRS increased from about 50 to about 200.

SBRT developed about a decade later than SRS but was based on similar principles. Swedish physicist Ingmar Lax and radiation oncologist Henric Blomgren, both at the Karolinska Hospital in Stockholm, were very familiar with the brain SRS procedures being carried out in their institution with the Gamma Knife. They reasoned that similar local control outcomes could be achieved at non-brain body sites with one or a few focally delivered fractions, even if targeting and immobilization issues for non-brain sites were more much complicated. They described their technique in 1994 (Lax et al. 1994) and in 1995 reported clinical outcomes in 31 patients with 42 malignant tumors of the liver, lung, or retroperitoneum, achieving local control in 80% of targets and prescribing at 50% isodose surface (Blomgren et al. 1995). David Larson visited the Karolinska Hospital in 1993 as an observer and brought their SBRT technique back to UCSF, where he treated 150 patients during 1993–1995. Thus, the origins of both SRS and SBRT can be traced in part to the Karolinska Hospital.

Standard Fractionation Versus Hypofractionation

Prominent pioneers of standard fractionation include French radiation oncologists Henri Coutard and Francois Baclesse, who treated laryngeal and breast cancers in Paris with various fractionation schemes lasting from 2 weeks to 10 months during the 1920s–1940s. They found that the uncomplicated control rate, often called the therapeutic ratio, peaked at 6–8 weeks, a result championed by Gilbert Fletcher in the USA following his training in Paris and confirmed by years of clinical experience throughout the world. In 1997, radiation oncologist Eli Glatstein stated: "Had Coutard and Baclesse not pioneered fractionation, radiotherapy probably would have fallen into oblivion due to the morbidities of single shot treatment. Indeed, much of the first half of this century was spent learning that doses large enough to sterilize a mass of tumor cells (10 logs) cannot be predictably given safely. Instead, fractionation evolved which permitted us to exploit repopulation, redistribution, reoxygenation, and repair."

Despite the above, clinicians have found that SRS- and SBRT-based hypofractionation techniques can be effectively and safely used for benign and malignant conditions in the brain and for initial or recurrent non-small cell lung cancer, prostate cancer, renal cell carcinoma, and hepatocellular cancer, and for oligometastases in the lung, liver, spine, and brain. To reconcile this with the established role of standard fractionation, one must recognize that with non-focal radiotherapy, the number of normal cells irradiated to full dose was historically as much as several logs *greater* than the number of tumor cells irradiated. However, with SRS and SBRT, the number of normal cells irradiated to full dose is as much as a log *less* than the number of tumor cells irradiated. If few normal tissue cells receive full dose, any clinically observable benefits of standard fractionation that are attributable to repopulation and repair are necessarily diminished. Similarly, the clinically observable fractionation benefits attributable to reoxygenation and redistribution within tumors are diminished if biological effective dose (BED) within the target can be increased safely.

For small tumors such as acoustic neuromas, meningiomas, and brain metastases, the reported uncomplicated control rate curve appears to be relatively flat over the range of 1–30 fractions. For some slightly larger targets, perhaps up to 3–5 cm in maximum dimension, the rates may peak at about five fractions, possibly because of the increased importance of reoxygenation and the increased volume of irradiated normal tissue with larger targets. Nevertheless, it is recognized that for many targets at CNS and non-CNS sites, the precise optimum fraction number with highly focal SRS or SBRT is not known, even though it is almost certainly far less than 30.

Summary

In summary, clinical results indicate that for carefully selected small targets of most histologies and at most anatomic body sites, favorable uncomplicated control rates can be achieved with 1–5 SRS or SBRT fractions, as the following chapters demonstrate. Nevertheless, physician judgment remains paramount, and in that context, it is appropriate to quote Professor Franz Buschke, ex-Chair of Radiation Oncology at UCSF, who wrote a letter to a referring physician in which he said, "Coutard taught us that the incidence of radiation sickness is related to the incompetence of the radiation therapist" (*Letter to a referring physician 1952*).

Nomenclature

The terms "SRS" and "SBRT," as used in this manual, apply to CNS and non-CNS anatomic sites, respectively, and in both cases involve delivery of a high biological effective dose (BED) in 1–5 fractions to small, focal, well-defined targets while minimizing nontarget dose. In the USA, this terminology is recognized by the American Medical Association (AMA) Current Procedural Terminology (CPT®) editorial panel, the AMA Specialty Society Relative Value Scale (RVS) Update Committee (RUC), the Centers for Medicare and Medicaid Services (CMS), and most commercial payers. Alternative nomenclature such as "SABR" ("stereotactic ablative radiotherapy" or "stereotactic ablative brain radiation" or "stereotactic ablative body radiotherapy") is favored by some clinicians and marketers but is not recognized by the CPT® editorial panel, RUC, or payers.

References

Benedict SH, Bova FJ, Clark B, Goetsch SJ, Hinson WH, Leavitt DD, et al. Anniversary paper: the role of medical physicists in developing stereotactic radiosurgery. Med Phys. 2008;35(9):4262–77.

Blomgren H, Lax I, Naslund I, Svanstrom R. Stereotactic high dose fraction radiation therapy of extracranial tumors using an accelerator. Clinical experience of the first thirty-one patients. Acta Oncol. 1995;34(6):861–70.

Kjelberg R. Isoeffective dose parameters for brain necrosis in relation to proton radiosurgical dosimetry. Stereotactic cerebral irradiation. INSERM symposium no 12: proceedings of the INSERM Symposium on Stereotactic Irradiations held in Paris (France), 13 July 1979. G. Szikla. Amsterdam; New York, New York, Elsevier/North-Holland Biomedical Press; sole distributors for the USA and Canada, North Holland: Elsevier; 1979. p. 157–66.

Lax I, Blomgren H, Naslund I, Svanstrom R. Stereotactic radiotherapy of malignancies in the abdomen. Methodological aspects. Acta Oncol. 1994;33(6):677–83.

Leksell L. The stereotaxic method and radiosurgery of the brain. Acta Chir Scand. 1951;102(4):316–9.

Lutz W, Winston K, Maleki N, Cassady R, Svensson G, Zervas N. Stereotactic radiation surgery in the brain using a 6 MV linear accelerator. Int J Radiat Oncol Biol Phys. 1984;10(Suppl 2):189.

Sturm V, Kober B, Höver KH, Schlegel W, Boesecke R, Pastyr O, Hartmann GH, Schabbert S, Zum Winkel K, Kunze S, et al. Stereotactic percutaneous single dose irradiation of brain metastases with a linear accelerator. Int J Radiat Oncol Biol Phys. 1987;13(2):279–82.

Part I
Physics of Stereotactic Radiosurgery and Stereotactic Body Radiotherapy

Chapter 2

Physics of Stereotactic Radiosurgery and Stereotactic Body Radiotherapy

Angélica Pérez-Andújar, Martina Descovich, and Cynthia Chuang

Pearls

- High doses of radiation delivered over 1–5 fractions (high biological effective dose).
- High-precision radiation delivery techniques combining image guidance solutions and stereotactic coordinate systems.
- Very conformal dose distribution with steep dose gradients.

A. Pérez-Andújar (✉)
Medical Physics, Memorial Sloan Kettering Cancer Center, West Harrison, NY, USA
e-mail: perezana@mskcc.org

M. Descovich
Division of Physics, Department of Radiation Oncology, University of California, San Francisco, San Francisco, CA, USA
e-mail: Martina.Descovich@ucsf.edu

C. Chuang
Radiation Oncology, Stanford University, Stanford, CA, USA
e-mail: chuangc@stanford.edu

© The Author(s), under exclusive license to Springer Nature Switzerland AG 2023
R. A. Sethi et al. (eds.), *Handbook of Evidence-Based Stereotactic Radiosurgery and Stereotactic Body Radiotherapy*,
https://doi.org/10.1007/978-3-031-33156-5_2

11

- Margin reduction, but consider that a large source of uncertainty relates to target delineation.
- Requires a rigorous quality assurance program and end-to-end commissioning procedures incorporating imaging, simulation, treatment planning, image guidance, motion management, and treatment delivery systems.
- Proton therapy is also used for stereotactic treatments, but the focus of this chapter will not be on particle therapy techniques. Some aspects were added to the chapter for completeness (ICRU 1998, 2007; Farr et al. 2021; Chang et al. 2016, 2017).

Basic Principles

- Originally developed for the treatment of intracranial lesions (Leksell 1983), radiosurgery is rapidly evolving.
- Both intracranial (SRS) and extracranial (SBRT) treatment sites.
- Recommendations for normal tissue dose tolerances are reported in AAPM TG 101 and several recent RTOG protocols (Benedict et al. 2010; Sperduto et al. 2013; Bezjak et al. 2019; Videtic et al. 2015; Lukka et al. 2018; Ryu et al. 2014).
- Table 2.1 presents general differences between conventional and SRS/SBRT treatments.

Patient setup and immobilization devices vary depending on body site, treatment platform, and capability of the delivery system to detect and correct for changes in patient position during treatment.

- SRS: Stereotactic head frame attached to the patient's skull using pins (Khan 2003). Frameless system could include thermoplastic mask with and without reflective markers. For SBRT: body frames, body cast, and vacuum bags could be used (Table 2.2).

TABLE 2.1 General comparison of conventional photon radiotherapy treatment versus stereotactic photon therapy (SRS/SBRT). Modified from Linda Hong's presentation (Benedict et al. 2010; Hong 2012)

Characteristic	Conventional RT	SRS/SBRT
Prescription dose per fraction	$\leq$3 Gy	$\geq$5 Gy
Number of fractions	$\geq$10	$\leq$5
Dose distribution	Homogeneous (max PTV dose ≈105–110%)	Heterogeneous (max PTV dose ≈110–200%)[a]
Dose gradient outside PTV	Shallow slope	Steep slope
Prescription isodose line	≈90–95%	≈50–95%[a]
Target definition	Tumor might not have a sharp boundary	Well-delineated target
PTV margin	≈cm	≈mm

[a] Heterogeneity of SRS/SBRT plans is highly dependent on the treatment technique used. The same applies to the prescription isodose lines

TABLE 2.2 Reported accuracy per body site for the commercially available SBRT immobilization devices (Taylor et al. 2011)

Site	Reported accuracy
Lung	1.8–5.0 mm
Liver	1.8–4.4 mm
Spine	1.0–3.0 mm

Location of the target has to be verified prior to beam on. Imaging techniques for SRS/SBRT treatment verification (Murphy et al. 2007; Herman et al. 2001; Broderick et al. 2007; Li et al. 2008; Jin et al. 2008):

- Orthogonal kV radiographs
- MV cone beam CT
- kV cone beam CT
- MV helical CT
- In-room diagnostic CT
- 4D-CBCT
- Infrared imaging
- Radiofrequency tracking
- Surface tracking

Management of respiratory motion for SBRT (lung, pancreas, liver, kidneys) (Keall et al. 2006) and motion encompassing techniques (4D-CT—ITV delineation):

- Abdominal compression—this method reduces the target excursion with breathing.
- Breath-hold—radiation is delivered when the patient is holding the breath.
- Gating—radiation is delivered only at a particular phase of respiration.
- Dynamic target tracking—beams are retargeted in real time to the continuously changing target position— advantages: no need for ITV expansion; no treatment interruptions; accounts for changes in target motion and respiratory pattern during treatment.

SRS/SBRT treatment parameters:

- Target volumes: The concepts of GTV, CTV, PTV, and ITV described in ICRU 50 and 62 for SRS also apply to SBRT planning (ICRU 1993a, b). PTV margins depend on body site, treatment device, localization technique, and imaging frequency. Typical margins range from 0 to 5 mm for SBRT treatments. The definition of the PTV for proton therapy systems included additional uncertainties like possible variations on the proton range. Margins could be defined per beam (ICRU 2007).

- Dose conformity: the high dose volume conforms tightly around the target.
- Dose heterogeneity: hot spots located within the target are often considered not only acceptable, but also desirable. The prescription dose is typically 50–90% of the maximum dose depending on the treatment delivery and treatment planning systems. Plans tend to be more homogenous for proton treatments.
- Dose gradient: the dose fall-off away from the target is steep. The volume of normal tissue receiving high doses of radiation is kept at a minimum. This is in comparison with other treatment techniques like 3D conformal.
- Beam energy: 6 MV photons offer the best compromise between beam penetration and penumbra characteristics. Many techniques use unflattened beams. 6 FFF and 10 FFF beams with high dose rates, 1400 MU/min and 2400 MU/min, respectively, are used to deliver the plan faster decreasing the probability of patient movement during treatment. For protons, the beam energy will depend on the delivery system, passive or active. Multiple beams with varying energies are used for active systems.
- Beam shaping: radiation is collimated to a small field using heavy metal cones (circular field 4–60 mm diameters), multileaf collimators (MLCs), or micro-MLCs (2.5 mm leaves' width). MLCs and micro-MLCs are used to deliver treatments developed with conformal beams, intensity-modulated fields, dynamic conformal arcs, volumetric modulated arcs, or a combination of these (ICRU 1993b). In the case of protons, compensator and range shifters could be used to shape the beam. The use of these will also depend on the delivery technique used (ICRU 1998).
- Treatments are delivered via coplanar and noncoplanar beam arrangements, and planar and noncoplanar arcs.

- Circular fields provide a sharper penumbra than micro-MLCs.
- Beam geometry: multiple nonoverlapping beams concentrically pointing to the target; 5–12 coplanar or noncoplanar beams; 1–4 coplanar or noncoplanar arcs; a continuously rotating fan beam; hundreds of noncoplanar pencil beams pointing to different parts of the target (non-isocentric beam arrangement) or to the same point (isocentric beam arrangement); the number of beams used in proton therapy will depend on the delivery technique, 2–3 for passive delivery, while for active systems, it will depend on the volume to be treated and the number of spots necessary to "fill up" that volume.

Plan optimization:

- Forward planning: the user manually adjusts beam arrangement, field shapes, and weights until the desirable dose distribution is achieved.
- Inverse planning: the user specifies plan objectives for target and normal structures, and a dose optimization algorithm calculates field shapes and weights based on the minimization of a mathematical cost function.
- Adaptive RT (ART) planning: treatment plans are adapted online to match patient anatomy using daily MRI scans acquired in treatment position.

Plan classification:

- 3-Dimensional conformal radiation therapy (3D-CRT): typically forward planned. It might be advantageous for moving targets, as the target is always in the open radiation field.
- Intensity-modulated radiation therapy (IMRT): typically inverse planned (although the field-in-field technique is forward planned). This also includes IMPT for protons.
- Arc therapy (RapidArc, VMAT).

Dose calculation algorithms:

- While the most accurate technique for dose calculation is Monte Carlo including for protons, convolution-superposition methods are sufficiently accurate in most clinical situations (Maes et al. 2018; Saini et al. 2018). Pencil beam algorithms (i.e., ray tracing) should only be used in homogeneous tissue. Pencil beam algorithms use simple radiological path length corrections to account for tissue heterogeneities and are largely inaccurate in low-density tissue. In these cases, heterogeneity corrections explicitly accounting for the transport of secondary electrons must be employed (Wilcox et al. 2010).
- Calculation grid: should be less than $2 \times 2 \times 2$ mm^3.

Treatment Platforms and Cross-Platform Comparisons

SRS/SBRT treatments can be performed using a variety of devices producing X-rays, gamma rays, or particle radiation (Tables 2.3 and 2.4) (ICRU 1998; Farr et al. 2021; Raaymakers et al. 2017; Mutic and Dempsey 2014; Combs et al. 2012; Dieterich and Gibbs 2011; Soisson et al. 2006; Choi et al. 2019; Paganelli et al. 2018; Cusumano et al. 2018; Kim et al. 2019; Gao et al. 2019; Pokhrel et al. 2021; Lim et al. 2019; Westover et al. 2012):

- Robotic linac radiosurgery system (CyberKnife)
- Helical TomoTherapy/Radixact
- Halcyon
- Gamma Knife
- MRI-guided systems/MR linacs
- Other linac-based systems
- Proton therapy

TABLE 2.3 Characteristics of various platforms for SRS/SBRT

Technology	Delivery system	Radiation	Dose rate	Beam shaping
CyberKnife	Compact linac mounted on a robotic arm	6 MV unflattened photon beam	Up to 1000 cGy/min	12 interchangeable tungsten cones; variable aperture collimator; MLC
TomoTherapy/Radixact	Helical, CT-like gantry equipped with a linac waveguide	6 MV unflattened photon beam	~850 cGy/min at isocenter	Binary MLC (64 leaves, 0.625 cm wide)
Halcyon	Ring-mounted 6 MV linac with a beam stopper	6 MV unflattened photon beam	~800 cGy/min at isocenter	Double-stacked and staggered MLC (total: 114, lower layer, two banks of 28 leaves each, upper layer, 2 banks of 29 leaves each, offset by 5 mm)
Gamma Knife	192 (Perfexion/Icon) ^{60}Co sources	1.17 and 1.33 MeV gamma rays	Initial source activity ~6000 ci, dose rate at focal point >3 Gy/min	Tungsten barrel subdivided into eight sectors (Perfexion)

MRI-guided systems (Elekta MRI-Linac)	Standing-wave linear accelerator	7 MV flattening filter free (FFF)	425 cGy/min	160 MLC (7.1 mm width) traveling in cranial-caudal direction. Field diaphragm perpendicular to the leaf travel direction
MRI-guided systems (MRIdian—View Ray)	Three 15,000-Ci ^{60}Co sources mounted on a ring gantry (120° apart) or linac	1.17 and 1.33 MeV gamma rays or 6 MV FFF photon energy	550–600 cGy/min	Each ^{60}Co head has independent doubly focused MLC system consisting of 30 leaf pairs (1.0–0.8 cm width)
Linac-based systems	Gantry-based linac rotating about the isocenter	Multiphoton energies (6, 10, 15, 18 MV flattened and unflattened) and electron energies	600 cGy/min up to 2400 cGy/min	MLC with standard (5 mm width) or micro (2.5 mm width) leaves
Protons	Synchrotron/cyclotron, synchro-cyclotron beam line treatment nozzle, rotating gantry	Depends on the technique, 2–3 beams passive delivery, multiple pencil beam energies for scanning systems, 60–250 MeV	Not applicable	Depending on the technique, beam collimators, compensators, and range shifters

(continued)

TABLE 2.3 (continued)

Technology	Field sizes	Beam arrangements	Treatment time
CyberKnife	Circular fields: 5–60 mm diameter MLC 10 × 12 cm	Hundreds of noncoplanar beams. No posterior beams	Long (hours: 20–50 min)
TomoTherapy/Radixact	Max field length 40 cm. Slice widths of 1, 2.5, and 5.0 cm	Treatments are delivered by synchronization of gantry rotation, couch translation, and MLC motion	Short (15–30 min)
Halcyon	28 cm × 28 cm (can extend with dual iso)	Multiple isocentric beams; coplanar arcs	Short (10–15 min)
Gamma Knife	4, 8, and 16 mm (Perfexion/ Icon); 4, 8, 14, 18 mm (models B-4C)	Multiple isocenters (shots)	Long (hours)
MRI-guided systems (Elekta MRI-Linac)	57.4 × 22.0 cm	Fixed coplanar beams, 3D conformal, and IMRT (arc therapy under investigation)	Long (hours: 15–30 min beam-on plus time required for ART)

MRI-guided systems (MRIdian — View Ray)	27.3×27.3 cm	Three fields to isocenter enabling delivery of 3D conformal and IMRT treatments	Long (hours: 30–50 min beam-on plus time required for ART)
Linac-based systems	Standard MLC typically gives a 40×40 field, micro-MLC gives a smaller field (12×14 cm^2)	Multiple isocentric beams; coplanar or noncoplanar beams; coplanar or noncoplanar arcs	Fast (15–30 min)
Protons	Depends on the technique, customized per patient and target volume	Depending on the technique, number of beams also depends on the techniques, coplanar and noncoplanar beams	Passive delivery fast 15 min, pencil beam scanning with gating ~45 min or more

TABLE 2.4 IGRT solutions

Technology	Imaging system	Imaging frequency	Image registration algorithms	Motion management
CyberKnife	2D orthogonal X-ray images at 45°	Every 15–150 s (typically 30–60 s)	Automatic registration of live camera images with DRR using site-specific algorithms (skull, fiducial, spine, lung)	Synchrony respiratory motion tracking
TomoTherapy/ Radixact	3D MVCT	Prior to each treatment	Automatic registration of MVCT with planning CT based on bony and/or soft tissue anatomical landmarks	Synchrony available on the Radixact platform
Halcyon	3D MVCT or 3D KV CBCT	Prior to each treatment	Automatic registration of CBCT with planning CT using either bony anatomy or soft tissue information	No fully automated deep inspiration breath-hold or phase-gated lung SBRT yet
Gamma Knife	CBCT available on the Icon	Prior to each treatment	Automatic registration of CBCT with planning CT using bony anatomy	Real-time infrared motion

MRI-guided systems (Elekta MRI-Linac)	1.5 T MRI	Online volumetric MRI: 3D SPGR, 3D balanced SSFP for patient monitoring every 7 s, cine-MRI	Online MRI registered with pretreatment images using deformable registration software	Gated delivery or MLC tracking combined with cine-MRI
MRI-guided systems (MRIdian—View Ray)	0.35 T MRI	Online volumetric MRI; fast 2D cine-MRI with interleaved sagittal/coronal slices	Deformable image registration with automatic contour propagation	Gated delivery (retracting ^{60}Co) verified by cine-MRI

(continued)

TABLE 2.4 (continued)

Technology	Imaging system	Imaging frequency	Image registration algorithms	Motion management
Linac-based systems	2D kV images, 2D fluoroscopy, 3D kV CBCT, 3D ultrasound, infrared system/surface imaging	Depending on imaging modality prior to or during treatment	Automatic registration of CBCT with planning CT using either bony anatomy or soft tissue information. 3D ultrasound images are also automatically co-registered to the planning CT	Gated delivery verified by 2D real-time fluoroscopic imaging or 4D-CBCT
Protons	Depends on the manufacturer, usually 2D kV images, 3D CBCT	Prior to each treatment, sometimes after treatment too	Automatic registration of CBCT, when available, with planning CT using either bony anatomy or soft tissue	Gated and self-gated available

Quality Assurance and Patient Safety

AAPM Task Group 101, Section VII.B., states that "*Specific tests should be developed to look at all aspects of the system both individually and in an integrated fashion*" (Benedict et al. 2010).

Systematic treatment accuracy verification is required for:

- CT/MR imaging
- Fusion uncertainties
- Planning calculation
- Target localization
- Dose delivery

This section focuses on target localization, IGRT system quality assurance, and dosimetry quality assurance.

Target localization accuracy:

- A top priority for SRS/SBRT treatments.
- The standard for target localization accuracy is the "Winston-Lutz" test or a similar test for frameless SRS/SBRT procedures (Solberg et al. 2008).
- Patient treatment target localization is achieved with either stereoscopic localization X-rays, volumetric imaging (CT, CBCT, MRI), or stereotactic head frames for Gamma Knife.

IGRT system quality assurance:

- Imaging isocenter and localization check (simple Winston-Luz) should be done daily when SRS/SBRT treatments are to be performed.

IGRT imaging systems:
Both kV-CBCT and MV-CBCT systems need:

- To be calibrated for proper registration of the treatment beam isocenter.
- To correct for accelerator and imaging component sags and flexes.
- To certify the geometric accuracy of the image-guided procedures (Bissonnette 2007; Bissonnette et al. 2008).

AAPM Task Group 142 on QA of Medical Accelerators, Table VI, recommends QA task tolerance and frequency for both planar and cone beam images. They include:

- ■ Safety and functionality
- ■ Geometrical accuracy:
  - ■ Imager isocenter accuracy
  - ■ 2D/2D match, 3D/3D registration accuracy
  - ■ Image magnification accuracy
  - ■ Imager isocenter accuracy with gantry rotation
- ■ Image quality:
  - ■ Contrast resolution and spatial resolution
  - ■ Hounsfield unit linearity and uniformity
  - ■ In-slice spatial linearity and slice thickness

For a detailed list of the recommended tests and tolerances, the reader is referred to TG 142 (Klein et al. 2009).

IGRT couch shift accuracy:

- ■ Need to verify the accuracy of the robotic couch movement:
  - ■ To ensure proper operation of the IGRT device and workflow.
  - ■ To assess communication between the image registration software and the remote-controlled couch.
  - ■ Is determined using the "residual correlation error" method (for details, please refer to TG 179).
  - ■ This value should be near 0 ± 2 mm, according to TG 179 (Bissonnette 2007).

Dosimetric Quality Assurance

Table 2.5 goes over the daily, monthly, and annual tests recommended for SRS and SBRT photon therapy systems based on TG 142 (Klein et al. 2009). Although many of these tests could be applicable to proton therapy, discussing the quality assurance aspects of particle therapy applications is out of the scope of this chapter. The AAPM Task Group TG 185 and TG 224 discuss the dosimetrical aspects of the quality assurance process for protons (Farr et al. 2021; Arjomandy

TABLE 2.5 Daily, monthly, and annual tests for SRS and SBRT photon therapy systems (recommendations based on TG 142) (Klein et al. 2009)

Daily QA	
Mechanical tests	**Tolerance**
Laser localization	1 mm
Optical distance indicator (ODI) @ iso	2 mm
Collimator size indicator	1 mm
Monthly QA	
Dosimetry tests	**Tolerance**
Dose rate output constancy	2% (@ stereo dose rate, MU)
Mechanical tests	**Tolerance**
Treatment couch position indicators	1 mm/0.5
Localizing lasers	$<\pm1$ mm
Annual QA	
Dosimetry tests	**Tolerance**
SRS arc rotation mode (range: 0.5–10 MU/deg)	Monitor unit set vs. delivered: 1.0 MU or 2% (whichever is greater) Gantry arc set vs. delivered: 1.0° or 2% (whichever is greater)
X-ray monitor unit linearity (output constancy)	$\pm5\%$ (2–4 MU) $\pm2\% \geqq5$ MU
Mechanical tests	**Tolerance**
Coincidence of radiation and mechanical isocenter	±1 mm from baseline
Stereotactic accessories, lockouts, etc.	Functional

et al. 2019). There are additional tests that should be performed for helical systems that are discussed in TG 148 (Langen et al. 2010).

A. Validation measurement vs. treatment planning output:
- Validation measurements need to be conducted after commissioning of the treatment planning system (TPS) and before the start of SRS/SBRT programs.
- These ensure that the TPS is calculating the correct dose, and the IGRT imaging system and the tracking/delivery system are delivering accurately.
- Performing an independent validation test of the delivered dose (for example by MD Anderson Phantom Laboratory) is strongly recommended.
- Validation measurements for photon beam systems include:
- Verify small field output factors using different types of detectors.
- Simple square field and/or circular cone outputs.
- Percent depth dose (PDD) and energy measurements compared with treatment planning calculations.
- Simple 3D plans and some IMRT plans should be planned, delivered, and measured to verify the dose calculation and delivery accuracy.
- Perform end-to-end tests covering the whole range of possible field size and IGRT methods (i.e., kV imaging, cone beam, for CK, different track algorithms).
- For multiple metastasis treatments, double- or multiple-isocenter plans would need to be verified.

- Special care should be taken to verify small field dosimetry during these SRS/SBRT end-to-end validation tests, since this particular area is most prone to commissioning inaccuracy and also dose planning uncertainty.

B. Routine quality assurance program:
- Routine quality assurance measurements are needed once the SRS/SBRT program has started to ensure the continuing dosimetry accuracy for these treatments.

C. Beam stability test:
  - The output and energy of the beam should be checked daily.
  - Tighter tolerance (constancy and accuracy to the sub-mm) is needed for SBRT/SRS treatments delivered using micro-MLC or high-definition MLC (Klein et al. 2009).
  - For CyberKnife robotic radiosurgery, TG 135 on "Quality assurance for robotic radiosurgery" recommends individual component QA and overall system QA, with specific daily, monthly, and annual frequency and tolerance tables in IVB, C, and D (Dieterich et al. 2011).
  - End-to-end test: including motion tracking/gating/breath-hold.
  - Each individual component of the SRS/SBRT process (imaging, localization, treatment delivery, etc.) has associated errors.
  - The cumulative system accuracy needs to be characterized through an end-to-end test using phantoms with measurement detectors and imaging on a routine basis.
  - For our CyberKnife system, end-to-end tests are conducted for all tracking modalities and collimator assemblies.
  - The end-to-end tests are performed monthly, and every time there is a repair or upgrade to the system.
D. Patient-specific QA:
  - Per TG 101, treatment-specific and patient-specific QA procedures should be established to govern both the treatment planning and delivery process as a whole, as well as to provide a sanity check of the setup.
  - Currently, published reports recommend performing patient-specific QA for every plan. However, there are ongoing efforts to reduce the number of patient plans needing QA.
  - Extremely small fields warrant patient-specific QA for all plans, since these cases involve both potential measurement uncertainty and positioning uncertainty:

- The output factors measured carried certain uncertainties (cones <7.5 mm and MLC fields <1 × 1 cm).
- Micro-MLC or Iris positioning uncertainties, examples:
  - CyberKnife: IRIS 10 mm or lower
  - For linac-based SRS/SBRT using micro-MLCs: any field size less than 1 cm
- Need to use equipment that has the correct resolution for QA, i.e., film for isodose distribution, diodes for dose profiles, pinpoint chamber, diode, or diamond detector for output factor measurements to avoid any volume averaging issues. For absolute dose measurement, use small-volume ion chambers (McEwen et al. 2014).

MRI-guided systems need (Kurz et al. 2020; Cho et al. 2017; Ahunbay et al. 2018; Weygand et al. 2016; Dorsch et al. 2019; Chen et al. 2020):

- Dedicated QA protocols for safe clinical operation
- To verify alignment of imaging and treatment isocenters using MR-compatible phantoms
- To account for effects of magnetic field on dose calculation
- To accurately measure absolute dose (point dose and 3D dose distribution) in the presence of magnetic field
- To check B-field homogeneity, signal-to-noise ratio, and spatial distortion induced by MRI
- To verify potential system interferences between linac and MRI
- To perform patient-specific QA on the adapted plan
- To perform comprehensive end-to-end tests for checking every step in the workflow, including image acquisition, image fusion, treatment plan adaptation, and treatment delivery

References

Ahunbay EE, Chen X, Paulson ES, Chen GP, Li A. An end-to-end verification of online adaptation process on a high-field MR-Linac. Int J Radiat Oncol Biol Phys. 2018;102(3):1.

Arjomandy B, Taylor P, Ainsley C, Safai S, Sahoo N, Pankuch M, et al. AAPM task group 224: comprehensive proton therapy machine quality assurance. Med Phys. 2019;46(8):e678–705.

Benedict SH, Yenice KM, Followill D, Galvin JM, Hinson W, Kavanagh B, et al. Stereotactic body radiation therapy: the report of AAPM task group 101. Med Phys. 2010;37(8):4078–101.

Bezjak A, Paulus R, Gaspar LE, Timmerman RD, Straube WL, Ryan WF, et al. Safety and efficacy of a five-fraction stereotactic body radiotherapy schedule for centrally located non-small-cell lung cancer: NRG oncology/RTOG 0813 trial. J Clin Oncol. 2019;37(15):1316–25.

Bissonnette JP. Quality assurance of image-guidance technologies. Semin Radiat Oncol. 2007;17(4):278–86.

Bissonnette JP, Moseley D, White E, Sharpe M, Purdie T, Jaffray DA. Quality assurance for the geometric accuracy of cone-beam CT guidance in radiation therapy. Int J Radiat Oncol Biol Phys. 2008;71(1 Suppl):S57–61.

Broderick M, Menezes G, Leech M, Coffey M, Appleyard R. A comparison of kilovoltage and megavoltage cone beam CT in radiotherapy. J Radiother Pract. 2007;6:173.

Chang JY, Jabbour SK, De Ruysscher D, Schild SE, Simone CB 2nd, Rengan R, et al. Consensus statement on proton therapy in early-stage and locally advanced non-small cell lung cancer. Int J Radiat Oncol Biol Phys. 2016;95(1):505–16.

Chang JY, Zhang X, Knopf A, Li H, Mori S, Dong L, et al. Consensus guidelines for implementing pencil-beam scanning proton therapy for thoracic malignancies on behalf of the PTCOG thoracic and lymphoma subcommittee. Int J Radiat Oncol Biol Phys. 2017;99(1):41–50.

Chen X, Ahunbay E, Paulson ES, Chen G, Li XA. A daily end-to-end quality assurance workflow for MR-guided online adaptive radiation therapy on MR-Linac. J Appl Clin Med Phys. 2020;21(1):205–12.

Cho JD, Park JM, Choi CH, Kim J, Wu H, S SP. Implementation of AAPM's TG-51 protocol on co-60 MRI-guided radiation therapy system. Prog Med Phys. 2017;28(4):7.

Choi CH, Kim JH, Kim JI, Park JM. Comparison of treatment plan quality among MRI-based IMRT with a linac, MRI-based IMRT with tri-co-60 sources, and VMAT for spine SABR. PLoS One. 2019;14(7):e0220039.

Combs SE, Ganswindt U, Foote RL, Kondziolka D, Tonn JC. State-of-the-art treatment alternatives for base of skull meningiomas: complementing and controversial indications for neurosurgery, stereotactic and robotic based radiosurgery or modern fractionated radiation techniques. Radiat Oncol. 2012;7:226.

Cusumano D, Dhont J, Boldrini L, Chiloiro G, Teodoli S, Massaccesi M, et al. Predicting tumour motion during the whole radiotherapy treatment: a systematic approach for thoracic and abdominal lesions based on real time MR. Radiother Oncol. 2018;129(3):456–62.

Dieterich S, Gibbs IC. The CyberKnife in clinical use: current roles, future expectations. Front Radiat Ther Oncol. 2011;43:181–94.

Dieterich S, Cavedon C, Chuang CF, Cohen AB, Garrett JA, Lee CL, et al. Report of AAPM TG 135: quality assurance for robotic radiosurgery. Med Phys. 2011;38(6):2914–36.

Dorsch S, Mann P, Elter A, Runz A, Spindeldreier CK, Kluter S, et al. Measurement of isocenter alignment accuracy and image distortion of an 0.35 T MR-Linac system. Phys Med Biol. 2019;64(20):205011.

Farr JB, Moyers MF, Allgower CE, Bues M, Hsi WC, Jin H, et al. Clinical commissioning of intensity-modulated proton therapy systems: report of AAPM task group 185. Med Phys. 2021;48(1):e1–e30.

Gao S, Netherton T, Chetvertkov MA, Li Y, Court LE, Simon WE, et al. Acceptance and verification of the halcyon-eclipse linear accelerator-treatment planning system without 3D water scanning system. J Appl Clin Med Phys. 2019;20(10):111–7.

Herman MG, Balter JM, Jaffray DA, McGee KP, Munro P, Shalev S, et al. Clinical use of electronic portal imaging: report of AAPM Radiation Therapy Committee Task Group 58. Med Phys. 2001;28(5):712–37.

Hong L, SBRT Treatment Planning: Practical Considerations American Association of Physicist in Medicine; AAPM Annual Meeting, 2012.

ICRU. Report 50: prescribing, recording, and reporting photon beam therapy. Bethesda MD: International Commission on Radiation Units and Measurements; 1993a.

ICRU. Report 62: prescribing, recording and reporting photon beam therapy (Supplement to ICRU Report 50). Bethesda MD: International Commission on Radiation Units and Measurements; 1993b.

ICRU. Report 59: clinical proton dosimetry part I: beam production. Beam delivery and measurement of absorbed dose. Bethesda, MD: International Commission on Radiation Units and Measurements; 1998.

ICRU. Report 78: prescribing, recording and reporting proton-beam therapy. Bethesda, MD: International Commission on Radiation Units and Measurements; 2007.

Jin JY, Yin FF, Tenn SE, Medin PM, Solberg TD. Use of the BrainLAB ExacTrac X-ray 6D system in image-guided radiotherapy. Med Dosim. 2008;33:124–34.

Keall PJ, Mageras GS, Balter JM, Emery RS, Forster KM, Jiang SB, et al. The management of respiratory motion in radiation oncology report of AAPM Task Group 76. Med Phys. 2006;33(10):3874–900.

Khan FM. The physics of radiation therapy. 3rd ed. Philadelphia: Lippincott Williams & Wilkins; 2003.

Kim H, Huq MS, Lalonde R, Houser CJ, Beriwal S, Heron DE. Early clinical experience with varian halcyon V2 linear accelerator: dual-isocenter IMRT planning and delivery with portal dosimetry for gynecological cancer treatments. J Appl Clin Med Phys. 2019;20(11):111–20.

Klein EE, Hanley J, Bayouth J, Yin FF, Simon W, Dresser S, et al. Task group 142 report: quality assurance of medical accelerators. Med Phys. 2009;36:4197–212.

Kurz C, Buizza G, Landry G, Kamp F, Rabe M, Paganelli C, et al. Medical physics challenges in clinical MR-guided radiotherapy. Radiat Oncol. 2020;15(1):93.

Langen KM, Papanikolaou N, Balog J, Crilly R, Followill D, Goddu SM, et al. QA for helical tomotherapy: report of the AAPM Task Group 148. Med Phys. 2010;37(9):4817–53.

Leksell L. Stereotactic radiosurgery. J Neurol Neurosurg Psychiatry. 1983;46:797–803.

Li G, Citrin D, Camphausen K, Mueller B, Burman C, Mychalczak B, et al. Advances in 4D medical imaging and 4D radiation therapy. Technol Cancer Res Treat. 2008;7(1):67–81.

Lim TY, Dragojević I, Hoffman D, Flores-Martinez E, Kim G. Characterization of the halcyon TM multileaf collimator system. J Appl Clin Med Phys. 2019;20(4):106–14.

Lukka HR, Pugh SL, Bruner DW, Bahary JP, Lawton CAF, Efstathiou JA, et al. Patient reported outcomes in NRG oncology RTOG 0938, evaluating two ultrahypofractionated regimens for prostate cancer. Int J Radiat Oncol Biol Phys. 2018;102(2):287–95.

Maes D, Saini J, Zeng J, Rengan R, Wong T, Bowen SR. Advanced proton beam dosimetry part II: Monte Carlo vs. pencil beam-based planning for lung cancer. Transl Lung Cancer Res. 2018;7(2):114–21.

McEwen M, DeWerd L, Ibbott G, Followill D, Rogers DW, Seltzer S, et al. Addendum to the AAPM's TG-51 protocol for clinical reference dosimetry of high-energy photon beams. Med Phys. 2014;41(4):041501.

Murphy MJ, Balter J, Balter S, BenComo JA Jr, Das IJ, Jiang SB, et al. The management of imaging dose during image-guided radiotherapy: report of the AAPM Task Group 75. Med Phys. 2007;34(10):4041–63.

Mutic S, Dempsey JF. The ViewRay system: magnetic resonance-guided and controlled radiotherapy. Semin Radiat Oncol. 2014;24(3):196–9.

Paganelli C, Whelan B, Peroni M, Summers P, Fast M, van de Lindt T, et al. MRI-guidance for motion management in external beam radiotherapy: current status and future challenges. Phys Med Biol. 2018;63(22):22TR03.

Pokhrel D, Visak J, Critchfield LC, Stephen J, Bernard ME, Randall M, et al. Clinical validation of ring-mounted halcyon linac for lung SBRT: comparison to SBRT-dedicated C-arm linac treatments. J Appl Clin Med Phys. 2021;22(1):261–70.

Raaymakers BW, Jurgenliemk-Schulz IM, Bol GH, Glitzner M, Kotte A, van Asselen B, et al. First patients treated with a 1.5 T MRI-Linac: clinical proof of concept of a high-precision, high-field MRI guided radiotherapy treatment. Phys Med Biol. 2017;62(23):L41–50.

Ryu S, Pugh SL, Gerszten PC, Yin FF, Timmerman RD, Hitchcock YJ, et al. RTOG 0631 phase 2/3 study of image guided stereotactic radiosurgery for localized (1-3) spine metastases: phase 2 results. Pract Radiat Oncol. 2014;4(2):76–81.

Saini J, Traneus E, Maes D, Regmi R, Bowen SR, Bloch C, et al. Advanced proton beam dosimetry part I: review and performance evaluation of dose calculation algorithms. Transl Lung Cancer Res. 2018;7(2):171–9.

Soisson ET, Tome WA, Richards GM, Mehta MP. Comparison of linac based fractionated stereotactic radiotherapy and tomotherapy treatment plans for skull-base tumors. Radiother Oncol. 2006;78(3):313–21.

Solberg TD, Medin PM, Mullins J, Li S. Quality assurance of immobilization and target localization systems for frameless stereotactic cranial and extracranial hypofractionated radiotherapy. Int J Radiat Oncol Biol Phys. 2008;71(1 Suppl):S131–5.

Sperduto PW, Wang M, Robins HI, Schell MC, Werner-Wasik M, Komaki R, et al. A phase 3 trial of whole brain radiation therapy and stereotactic radiosurgery alone versus WBRT and SRS with temozolomide or erlotinib for non-small cell lung cancer and 1 to 3 brain metastases: Radiation Therapy Oncology Group 0320. Int J Radiat Oncol Biol Phys. 2013;85(5):1312–8.

Taylor ML, Kron T, Franich RD. A contemporary review of stereotactic radiotherapy: inherent dosimetric complexities and the potential for detriment. Acta Oncol. 2011;50(4):483–508.

Videtic GM, Hu C, Singh AK, Chang JY, Parker W, Olivier KR, et al. A randomized phase 2 study comparing 2 stereotactic body radiation therapy schedules for medically inoperable patients with stage I peripheral non-small cell lung cancer: NRG oncology RTOG 0915 (NCCTG N0927). Int J Radiat Oncol Biol Phys. 2015;93(4):757–64.

Westover KD, Seco J, Adams JA, Lanuti M, Choi NC, Engelsman M, et al. Proton SBRT for medically inoperable stage I NSCLC. J Thorac Oncol. 2012;7(6):1021–5.

Weygand J, Fuller CD, Ibbott GS, Mohamed AS, Ding Y, Yang J, et al. Spatial precision in magnetic resonance imaging-guided radiation therapy: the role of geometric distortion. Int J Radiat Oncol Biol Phys. 2016;95(4):1304–16.

Wilcox EE, Daskalov GM, Lincoln H, Shumway RC, Kaplan BM, Colasanto JM. Comparison of planned dose distributions calculated by Monte Carlo and ray-trace algorithms for the treatment of lung tumors with cyberknife: a preliminary study in 33 patients. Int J Radiat Oncol Biol Phys. 2010;77(1):277–84.

Part II
Clinical Applications

Chapter 3
Intracranial Tumors

Matthew S. Susko, Jessica Chew, Steve E. Braunstein, David A. Larson, and David R. Raleigh

M. S. Susko · J. Chew · S. E. Braunstein
Department of Radiation Oncology, University of California, San Francisco, San Francisco, CA, USA
e-mail: Matthew.Susko@ucsf.edu; Jessica.Chew@ucsf.edu; BraunsteinSE@radonc.ucsf.edu

D. A. Larson
(deceased), Departments of Radiation Oncology and Neurological Surgery, University of California, San Francisco, San Francisco, CA, USA
e-mail: david.larson@ucsf.edu

D. R. Raleigh (✉)
Departments of Radiation Oncology and Neurological Surgery, University of California, San Francisco, San Francisco, CA, USA
e-mail: David.Raleigh@ucsf.edu

© The Author(s), under exclusive license to Springer Nature Switzerland AG 2023
R. A. Sethi et al. (eds.), *Handbook of Evidence-Based Stereotactic Radiosurgery and Stereotactic Body Radiotherapy*, https://doi.org/10.1007/978-3-031-33156-5_3

39

Pearls

Brain Metastases

- Most common intracranial tumor (20–40% of all cancer patients on autopsy); most commonly from lung cancer, breast cancer, or melanoma.
- "Solitary" metastasis: one brain lesion as the only site of disease; "single" metastasis: one brain metastasis, other sites of disease
- Start dexamethasone up to 4 mg q6hrs for neurologic symptoms; no role for steroids in asymptomatic patients. Taper as tolerated once radiotherapy is complete; no evidence for seizure prophylaxis (Table 3.1).
- Prognostic factors include KPS, age, number of brain metastases, and tumor histopathologic characteristics.

Meningioma

- Thirty percent of primary intracranial neoplasms; twofold more likely in women (though with equal incidence rates for anaplastic meningiomas).

TABLE 3.1 RTOG RPA for brain metastases (Gaspar et al. 1997)

Class	Characteristics	Survival (months)
I	KPS 70–100	7.1
	Age < 65	
	Primary tumor controlled	
	Metastases to brain only	
II	All others	4.2
III	KPS <70	2.3

TABLE 3.2 Simpson grading system for meningioma resection

Grade I	Macroscopic complete removal with excision of dural attachment, any abnormal bone, and involved venous sinus(es)
Grade II	Macroscopic complete removal with coagulation of dural attachment
Grade III	Macroscopic complete removal of intradural component(s), without resection or coagulation of dural attachment or extradural extensions
Grade IV	Partial removal with residual intradural tumor in situ
Grade V	Simple decompression with or without biopsy

Pathogenesis linked to ionizing radiation, viral infection, sex hormones, NF2, and loss of chromosome 22q.

- Radiosurgery utilized for definitive treatment of WHO grade 1 meningiomas or for adjuvant therapy after subtotal resection (Table 3.2).

Acoustic Neuroma

- Acoustic neuromas (i.e., vestibular schwannomas) arise from myelin sheath Schwann cells surrounding the vestibular nerve; 6–8% of intracranial tumors, overall incidence ~1% on autopsy studies.
- Risk factors include acoustic trauma and coincidence with parathyroid adenoma; bilateral acoustic neuromas pathopneumonic for NF2.
- Both CN VII and VIII may be affected. Symptomatic presentation with hearing loss, tinnitus, vertigo, and unsteady gait. Extension into the cerebellopontine angle may lead to dysfunction of CN V (trigeminal

pain) and the facial nerve (facial paresis and taste disturbances), as well as compression of the posterior fossa (ataxia, hydrocephalus, and death).
- Mean growth rate ~ 2 mm per year, although may remain stable for years.

Paraganglioma

- Rare neuroendocrine tumors with incidence of ~1:1,000,000; sometimes called glomus tumors or chemodectomas as they arise from glomus cells which function as chemoreceptors along blood vessels.
- Can occur in the abdomen (85%), thorax (12%), and the head and neck (3%); usually benign (<5% malignant potential).

Pituitary Adenoma

- Approximately 10% of intracranial tumors (5–25% incidence on autopsy), almost all of which arise in the anterior lobe; 75% functional (30–50% prolactinoma, 25% GH, 20% ACTH, and <1% TSH).
- Microadenoma <1 cm; macroadenoma ≥1 cm.
- Presenting symptoms include headaches, bitemporal hemianopsia and/or loss of color discrimination from optic chiasm compression, hydrocephalus from third ventricle obstruction, and cranial nerve palsies with extension to the cavernous sinus.
- Forbes-Albright syndrome from prolactinoma: amenorrhea-galactorrhea in women, impotence and infertility in men.
- Both mass effect and radiation damage to the pituitary infundibulum can cause an elevation in prolactin due to loss of hypothalamic inhibition ("stalk effect").

- Hormone levels typically normalize within 1–2 years after radiotherapy.

Arteriovenous Malformation (AVM)

- Abnormal congenital communication between arterial and venous vasculature at a "nidus"; supraphysiologic hydrodynamic gradient.
- Low incidence in the US population (0.14%), but 8% coincidence with cerebral aneurysm.
- Annual rate of spontaneous hemorrhage ~2–6%, with morbidity 20–30% and mortality 10–15% per event; after angiographic obliteration, lifetime risk of hemorrhage ≤1%.
- SRS induces vascular wall hyperplasia and luminal thrombosis, but requires several years to achieve full effect.
- AVMs differ from cavernous malformations insofar as the latter are composed of sinusoidal vessels without a large feeding artery, and therefore have a low-pressure gradient (Table 3.3).

TABLE 3.3 Spetzler-Martin AVM grading system (total score 1–5)

Size of nidus	<3 cm = 1
	3–6 cm = 2
	>6 cm = 3
Location	Adjacent to non-eloquent brain = 0
	Adjacent to eloquent cortex = 1
Venous drainage	Superficial = 0
	Deep = 1

Neuropathic Facial Pain

Trigeminal Neuralgia

- CN V sensory nucleus disorder resulting in episodic, provokable (i.e., shaving, brushing teeth, wind, etc.), paroxysmal, unilateral, severe, lancinating pain lasting seconds to minutes in the distribution of the trigeminal nerve.
- Predominantly idiopathic, although may be the result of trigeminal nerve compression by an aberrant artery or vein, or demyelination due to multiple sclerosis. Secondary trigeminal neuralgia can develop due to mass effect from meningioma, vestibular schwannoma, AVM, aneurysm, or other lesions.
- Diagnosis of exclusion; obtain MRI to rule out cerebellopontine angle neoplasm.
- Median time to pain relief after SRS is ~1 month; 50–60% CR, 15–20% PR; <10% incidence of facial numbness after treatment.

Cluster Headache

- Sudden onset of unilateral pain typically along the distribution of CN V1; associated with ipsilateral autonomic activity including ptosis, meiosis, lacrimation, conjunctival injection, rhinorrhea, and nasal congestion.
- Etiology unclear; 6:1 male to female predominance.
- GKRS to the trigeminal nerve alone not successful and is associated with much higher rate of toxicity than during SRS for trigeminal neuralgia (Donnet et al. 2006; McClelland et al. 2006). Investigation of SRS to the pterygopalatine ganglion +/− trigeminal nerve root is ongoing (Kano et al. 2011; Lad et al. 2007).

Sphenopalatine Neuralgia (Sluder's Neuralgia)

- Rare craniofacial pain syndrome with 2:1 female predominance associated with unilateral pain in the orbit, mouth, nose, and posterior mastoid process as well as ipsilateral autonomic stimulation from vasomotor activity.
- Etiology unclear, though potentially related to pterygopalatine ganglion irritation from inflammation/infection of the sphenoid or posterior ethmoid sinuses.
- Radiosurgical data limited to case reports of sphenopalatine ganglion treatment (Pollock and Kondziolka 1997).

Other

- Small retrospective series of SRS for residual/recurrent pineal parenchymal tumors, craniopharyngiomas, and neurocytomas with high long-term local control and survival.
- SRS used as salvage treatment for certain functional disorders, including epilepsy, Parkinson disease, and essential tremor with varying efficacy.
- Stereotactic treatment of residual/recurrent glial tumors, medulloblastoma, and other aggressive CNS malignancies has been reported, but outcomes are discouraging. Hypofractionation of recurrent glial tumors is effective as salvage.

Treatment Indications

- In general, SRS+WBRT is associated with longer survival than WBRT alone in patients with single metastases and KPS ≥70, improved LC and KPS preservation in patients with 1–4 metastases and KPS

≥70, and potentially, improved survival in patients with KPS <70.

- SRS alone may provide equivalent survival and LC, plus improved neurocognitive outcomes when compared to SRS + WBRT or WBRT alone in patients with ≤3 metastases; close surveillance and salvage treatment are essential.
- After resection, both SRS+WBRT and WBRT alone are acceptable adjuvant strategies, although SRS alone may be used in select cases with minimal intracranial disease and close surveillance (Linskey et al. 2010) (Tables 3.4 and 3.5).

TABLE 3.4 Radiosurgical treatment indications for brain metastases

Single lesion	Surgical resection + SRS to cavity
RPA class I–II	SRS alone for medically/surgically inoperable cases
2–4 Lesions	SRS +/− surgical resection with excellent prognosis/KPS
RPA class I–II	
KPS ≤60, extensive intracranial/extracranial disease, and in combination with SRS as described above	WBRT

TABLE 3.5 Radiosurgical treatment indications for benign intracranial neoplasms

Meningioma	• Recurrent/residual disease after surgery
	• Recurrent disease after prior SRS/RT
	• Medically or surgically inoperable
Acoustic neuroma	• STR (LF 45% without adjuvant RT vs. 6% with postoperative SRS)
	• Patient desire for greater preservation of useful hearing (30–50% with surgery)
Pituitary adenoma	• Adjuvant therapy after STR of macroadenoma with persistent postoperative hypersecretion or residual suprasellar extension
	• Consider medical management with bromocriptine or cabergoline for prolactin-secreting microadenoma
	• Medically inoperable, surgically inaccessible, or anticipated high morbidity due to Spetzler-Martin grade
Neurofacial pain	• Failure of medical management (carbamazepine, phenytoin, gabapentin, baclofen, etc.)
	• Failure of surgical management (radiofrequency rhizotomy, balloon compression, microvascular decompression, etc.)

Workup

- H&P with emphasis on neurologic components.
- Review of systems including any sensory changes, neurologic symptoms, and endocrine abnormalities.
- Laboratories:
  - No routine serum tests necessary for the evaluation of brain metastases, meningioma, AVM, neurofacial pain syndromes, etc.
  - Acoustic neuroma: Audiometry is the best initial screening and typically shows sensorineural hearing loss (as will the Rinne and Weber tests).
  - Pituitary adenomas: Endocrine evaluation with prolactin, basal GH, serum ACTH, free cortisol, dexamethasone suppression, TSH, T3, T4, FSH, LH, plasma estradiol, and testosterone levels.
- Imaging:

  - Thin-cut MRI with T1 pre- and post-gadolinium, T2, and FLAIR (fluid attenuation inversion recovery) sequences; tumor enhancement after gadolinium correlates with breakdown of the blood–brain barrier, abnormal T2 signal indicative of gliosis and/or edema.
  - Can consider increased dose gadolinium at the time of radiosurgery to improve sensitivity of detection of brain metastases.
  - Hemorrhagic metastases most often seen with renal cell cancer, choriocarcinoma, and melanoma.
  - Magnetic resonance spectroscopy: tumors characterized by increased choline (cellularity marker), decreased *N*-acetylaspartic acid (NAA; neuronal marker), and decreased creatinine (cellular energy marker); necrosis associated with increased lactate (anaerobic metabolism), and decreased choline/NAA/creatinine.
  - Dynamic magnetic resonance perfusion: relative cerebral blood flow (CBV) elevated in tumors

(often in concert with grade), and decreased in areas of radiation necrosis and tumefactive demyelination.

- Postoperative MRI should be performed within 48 h of surgery to document residual disease; acute blood appears as increased intrinsic T1 signal pre-contrast.
- "Dural tail sign" can be indicative of either tumor extension or vascular congestion associated with tumors adjacent or intrinsic to the meninges (seen with 60% of meningiomas).
- Meningiomas are isointense on T1 and T2 and intensely enhance with gadolinium; evidencc of bony destruction or hyperostosis in 15–20% of cases. Acoustic neuroma: seen as enhancing "ice cream cone" in the internal acoustic canal or as "dumbbell" projecting into the foramen magnum.
- Pituitary adenomas: X-ray skeletal survey should be performed in cases of acromegaly to evaluate growth plates.
- AVM: Co-registration of cerebral angiography and time of flight MRI sequences helpful for target delineation.
- Neuropathic facial pain: Thin slice (1 mm) MRI/MRA has sensitivity and specificity of 89% and 50%, respectively, for identifying vascular compression of the trigeminal nerve.

Radiosurgical Technique

- Simulation and treatment planning.
    - Simulation with stereotactic frame or mask depending on treatment modality.
    - Primary MRI planning with thin cuts (1–2 mm) preferred for intracranial radiosurgery, with fusion of preoperative scans if available.

- If necessary, CT slices no thicker than 2 mm should be obtained and co-registered with MRI images.
- Target volumes:
  - Brain metastases: GTV alone for intact lesions. For resection cavities, a 1–2 mm margin may increase local control (Soltys et al. 2008). Consensus guidelines recommend 5–10 mm expansion along the dura underlying the bone flap to account for microscopic disease.
  - Meningioma, acoustic neuroma, pituitary adenoma, and other benign intracranial tumors: GTV with 0–2 mm margin depending on degree of immobilization and stereotaxis.
  - Trigeminal neuralgia: Target ipsilateral trigeminal nerve adjacent to the pons in the retrogasserian cistern with a single, 4 mm shot. Retreatment isocenter should be located 2–3 mm away from initial target if possible.
- Dose prescription:
  - See Table 3.6.
  - Consider hypofractionation in select cases if dose constraints to critical structures cannot be met with single-fraction treatment.
- Dose delivery.
  - Multiple treatment modalities available, but most centers employ GK SRS, frameless robotic radiosurgery, and/or linac-based SRS.

TABLE 3.6 Dose recommendations and outcomes for intracranial stereotactic radiosurgery

Presentation	Recommended dose	Outcomes
Brain metastases	• 13–24 Gy/1 fraction depending on tumor volume/location	
	• Dose reduction or hypofractionation (21–30 Gy/3–5 fractions) with larger lesions and/or resection cavities	
	• Consider dose reduction (15–16 Gy) for brainstem lesions	
Meningioma	• Individualize dose based on tumor volume/location/ surgical/radiosurgical history	
	• 15 Gy/1 fraction for WHO grade I–III lesions; hypofractionation to 25–30 Gy/5 fractions possible, although long-term results unknown (UCSF experience). • Grade III lesions may require higher dose	Long-term LC >90% for WHO grade I lesions

(continued)

TABLE 3.6 (continued)

Presentation	Recommended dose	Outcomes
Acoustic neuroma	• 12–13 Gy/1 fraction	LC and preservation of CNs V and VII in excess of 95%; hearing preservation ~75%
	• 18–25 Gy/3–5 fractions	Appears safe and effective, but long-term results are unknown
Paraganglioma	• 15 Gy/1 fraction or hypofractionation to 25 Gy/5 fractions	LC ~100%
Pituitary adenoma	• Nonfunctioning tumors: 12–20 Gy/1 fraction	
	• Functioning tumors: 15–30 Gy/1 fraction (maximal safe dose); discontinue medical therapy 4 weeks prior to radiosurgery.	
	• Single-fraction optic apparatus tolerance: 8 Gy	
	• 21–25 Gy/3–5 fractions	Appears safe and effective, but long-term results unknown

(continued)

TABLE 3.6 (continued)

Presentation	Recommended dose	Outcomes
AVM	• Individualize dose based on tumor volume; staged radiosurgery for larger lesions	2-Year obliteration rate for single-fraction treatment: <2 cm 90–100%, >2 cm 50–70%
	• 18 Gy/1 fraction for 8 cm^3 target(s); dose escalation when feasible and safe (UCSF experience)	
Trigeminal neuralgia	• Primary: 70–90 Gy (100% isodose line)	Pain relief in ~30–80% of patients, although retreatment common; dose related to both relief from symptoms and development of new symptoms
	• Retreatment: 50–70 Gy (100% isodose line)	
Pineal tumors	• Fractioned neuraxial RT for high-grade lesion; 15 Gy SRS reserved for residual tumor or local recurrence after RT	

Toxicities and Management

- Stereotactic frame:
  - Mild headache immediately following frame removal, usually subsiding within 60 min.
  - Minimal bleeding from pin insertion sites requiring compression.
  - Peri-orbital edema resolving with head elevation and warm compress.
  - <1% Risk of superficial skin infection.
- Acute (1 week to 6 months):
  - Alopecia and skin changes following treatment of superficial lesions.
  - Mild fatigue.
  - Transient worsening of neurologic symptoms due to edema potentially requiring steroids.
- Late (>6 months):

  - Radiation necrosis: Overall five-percent rate of symptomatic brain necrosis after SRS; typically resolves with steroids, but may require surgical intervention.
  - Endocrine abnormalities.
  - Cranial nerve dysfunction following treatment of skull base tumors.
  - Rare: memory impairment and cavernous malformations.
  - Isolated case reports of stroke, facial palsy/hyperesthesia, vision loss, and eye dryness after SRS for trigeminal neuralgia, all of which are very rare.

Recommended Follow-Up

- Brain metastases and other high-grade lesions:
  - MRI 4–12 weeks after treatment, then every 2–3 months for the first 2-years, followed by imaging

every 6 months for the next 3 years, and yearly thereafter; imaging intervals should be individualized according to clinical symptoms and lesion trajectory.

- Low-grade lesions (meningioma, acoustic neuroma, paraganglioma, etc.):
  - MRI every 6–12 months for the first 2-years, then annually; imaging intervals should be individualized according to clinical symptoms and lesion trajectory.
- Pituitary adenoma and other peri-sellar lesions:
  - Endocrine testing every 6–12 months with visual field testing annually.
- Acoustic neuromas and cerebellopontine angle tumors:
  - Formal audiometry annually.
- AVM:
  - MRI up to once per year for 3 years after treatment, with angiogram to confirm response after 3 years.
- Neuropathologic facial pain and functional disorders:

  - Clinical follow-up only.

Evidence

Brain Metastases

SRS Boost with WBRT

- RTOG 95-08 (Andrews et al. 2004): Randomized, multi-institution trial including 333 patients with 1–3 brain metastases and KPS ≥70 treated with WBRT (37.5 Gy/15 fractions) plus SRS (15–24 Gy/1 fraction) vs. WBRT alone. Significant survival advantage with SRS in patients with a single metastasis on univariate analysis (6.5 vs. 4.9 months), RPA class I on multivariate analysis (11.6 vs. 9.6 months), and trends for advantage with lung histology (5.9 vs. 3.9 months), and tumor size >2 cm (6.5 vs. 5.3 months). WBRT+SRS also associated with significantly higher 1-year LC (82% vs. 71%), and improved KPS (13% vs. 4%) with decreased steroid use at 6 months. Minimal acute- and long-term toxicity.

■ University of Pittsburgh (Kondziolka et al. 1999a, b): Randomized trial of 27 patients with 2–4 brain metastases and KPS ≥70 treated with WBRT (30 Gy/12 fractions) plus SRS (16 Gy/1 fraction) vs. WBRT alone. Study stopped early due to significant interim benefit in LC for WBRT+SRS (100% vs. 8%); median time to LF 6 months with WBRT vs. 36 months with WBRT+SRS. No difference in OS (8 vs. 11 months), and survival equal (~11 months) when accounting for SRS salvage in WBRT arm. No difference in OS or LC depending on histological type, number of brain metastases, or extent of extracranial disease.

SRS Alone or With WBRT

■ RTOG 90-05 (Shaw et al. 2000): Dose escalation study including 156 patients (36% recurrent primary brain tumors, median prior dose of 60 Gy; 64% recurrent brain metastases, median prior dose of 30 Gy). Maximum tolerated doses of 24 Gy, 18 Gy, and 15 Gy for tumors ≤20 mm, 21–30 mm, and 31–40 mm in diameter, respectively; MTD for tumors <20 mm likely higher, but investigators reluctant to escalate further. Tumor diameter ≥2 cm significantly associated with increasing risk of grade ≥3 neurotoxicity on multivariate analysis; higher dose and KPS also associated with greater neurotoxicity. Actuarial 24-month risk of radionecrosis 11%. Patients with primary brain tumors and those treated on linear accelerators (as opposed to GKRS) had ~2.8-fold greater chance of local progression.

■ JROSG 99-1 (Aoyama et al. 2006): Randomized, multi-institution trial including 132 patients with 1–4 brain metastases (diameter < 3 cm) and KPS ≥70, treated with SRS (18–25 Gy/1 fraction) vs. WBRT (30 Gy/10 fractions) followed by SRS. Trial stopped early due to low probability of detecting a difference between arms. Addition of WBRT reduced rate of new metastases (64% vs. 42%) and need for salvage brain treatment, and improved 1-year recurrence rate (47% vs. 76%). No difference in OS (~8 months), neurologic or KPS preservation, or MMSE score.

- MDACC (Chang et al. 2009): Randomized trial including 58 patients with 1–3 brain metastases and KPS ≥70 treated with SRS (15–24 Gy/1 fraction) vs. SRS + WBRT (30 Gy/12 fractions) and followed with formal neurocognitive testing. Trial stopped early due to significant decline in memory and learning at 4 months with WBRT by Hopkins Verbal Learning Test (52% vs. 24%). However, WBRT also associated with improved LC (100% vs. 67%) and distant brain control (73% vs. 45%) at 1 year. Significantly longer OS with SRS alone (15 vs. 6 months), but patients in this arm received more salvage therapy including repeat SRS (27 vs. 3 retreatments).

- UCSF (Sneed et al. 1999): Retrospective review of GKRS (*n* = 62) vs. GKRS+WBRT (*n* = 43); treatment characteristics individualized according to physician preference. OS (~11 months) and 1-year local FFP (71% vs. 79%) equivalent. Although brain FFP significantly worse for SRS alone (28% vs. 69%), no difference when allowing for first salvage (62% vs. 73%) after 1 year.

- Sneed et al. (2002): Retrospective, multi-institution review of 569 patients with brain metastases treated with SRS alone (*n* = 268) vs. WBRT+SRS (*n* = 301); exclusion criteria included resection of brain metastasis and interval from end of WBRT to SRS >1 month. Median and overall survival no different among respective RPA statuses (I: 14 vs. 15 months; II: 8 vs. 7 months; class III: ~5 months). Twenty-four percent WBRT salvage rate in SRS patients.

- EORTC 22951-26001 (Kocher et al. 2011): Randomized, multi-institution trial of WBRT (*n* = 81, 30 Gy/10 fractions) vs. observation (n = 79) following either surgery or SRS for 1–3 brain metastases in patients with stable systemic disease and ECOG performance status 0–2. Median time to ECOG performance status deterioration >2: 10 months with observation and 9.5 months with WBRT. OS similarly equivalent (~11 months), although WBRT reduced 2-year relapse at both new and initial sites. Salvage therapies used more frequently in the observation arm.

- University of Cologne (Kocher et al. 2004): Retrospective review of patients with 1–3 previously untreated cerebral metastases treated with linac-based SRS (n = 117, median dose 20 Gy/1 fraction) or WBRT (n = 138, 30–36 Gy/10 fractions) stratified by RPA class. Rate of salvage WBRT: SRS group 22%, WBRT group 7%. Significantly longer survival after SRS in RPA class I (25 vs. 5 months) and class II (6 vs. 4 months) patients; no difference in RPA class III patients (4 vs. 2.5 months).

- NCCTG (Brown et al. 2016): Prospective phase III trial randomizing participants to SRS alone or SRS plus WBRT for 1–3 brain metastases with primary endpoint of neurocognitive deterioration at 3 months. Overall 213 participants showed less cognitive deterioration at 3 months after SRS alone (63.5%) compared to SRS and WBRT (91.7%) $p < 0.001$. Time to intracranial failure was significantly shorter for SRS alone (HR 3.6; $p < 0.001$), with no significant difference in OS at 10.4 months for SRS alone and 7.4 months for SRS plus WBRT ($p = 0.92$).

SRS for >4 Brain Metastases

- University of Pittsburgh (Bhatnagar et al. 2006): Retrospective review of 105 patients with ≥4 brain metastases (median 5, range 4–18) treated with single-session GKRS (median marginal dose 16 Gy/1 fraction) plus WBRT (46%), after failure of WBRT (38%), or alone (17%). Median OS 8 months (RPA class I: 18 months, class II: 9 months, and class III: 3 months), 1-year LC 71%, and median time to progression or new brain metastases 9 months. Total treatment volume, age, RPA classification, and median marginal dose (but not the total number of metastases treated) are all significant prognostic factors on multivariate analysis.

■ JLGK0901 (Yamamoto et al. 2014): Prospective observational cohort of 1194 patients treated with SRS to 1–10 brain metastases, analyzed by number of metastases (1, 2–4, and 5–10). Median OS for 1 brain metastasis 13.9 months, 2–4 metastases 10.8 months, 5–10 metastases 10.8 months, with non-inferiority being demonstrated between SRS treatment of 5–10 lesions compared to 2–4 ($p < 0.0001$ uskom for non-inferiority). No significant difference demonstrated the number of treatment related adverse events in either group with multiple brain metastases ($p = 0.89$).

SRS Boost After Resection

■ Stanford (Soltys et al. 2008): Retrospective review of 76 resection cavities treated with SRS (median marginal dose 18.6 Gy, mean target volume 9.8 cm^3). Actuarial LC at 6 and 12 months: 88 and 79%, respectively. Conformality index significantly correlated with improved LC on univariate analysis; LC 100% for the least conformal quartile, and 63% for all others. Target volume, dose, and number of fractions are not significant. Recommendation for 2 mm margin around resection cavities.

■ NCCTG N107C (Brown et al. 2017): Prospective phase III trial of patients with resected brain metastasis randomized to SRS versus WBRT, primary outcomes were neurocognitive deterioration free survival and OS. Accrued 194 patients with median follow-up of 11.1 months (IQR 5.1-18), SRS associated with less frequent neurocognitive decline at 6 months (52% vs. 85%; p = 0.00031), with no significant difference in OS between the two groups (12.2 m vs. 11.6 m; p = 0.70).

- MDACC (Mahajan et al. 2017): Single-institution phase III trial of 132 patients randomized to postoperative SRS versus observation for 1–3 resected brain metastases. Median follow-up of 11·1 months (IQR 4·8-20·4) with 12-month FFLR of 43% (95% CI 31–59) for the observation group and 72% (60–87) for the SRS with HR 0·46 [95% CI 0·24–0·88]; p = 0·015) favoring SRS. No significant difference in OS was seen between observation and SRS (HR 1.26; 95% CI 0·84–1·98).

- Soliman et al. (2018): Expert consensus guidelines for target delineation of postoperative surgical cavity, using ten example clinical scenarios. High level of agreement between experts with recommendation for inclusion of the entire surgical tract, extension of CTV 5–10 mm along overlaying dura due to risk of microscopic disease, ≤5 mm extension into venous sinus when there is preoperative contact.

Brainstem Lesions

- Chen et al. (2021): Systematic review and comparative meta-analysis of SRS to brainstem metastases. Inclusive of 32 retrospective studies comprising 1446 patients with 1590 brainstem metastases treated to a median marginal dose of 16 Gy (range 6–39 Gy) in a median of 1 (range 1–13) fractions. Rate of local control at 1-year was 86% (95% CI 83–88%), with symptomatic improvement in 55% (95% CI 47–63%), and OS at 1-year was 33% (95% CI 30–37%). Toxicity of any grade was found in 5.6% of patients, with 2.4% (95% CI 1.5–3.7%) developing grade 3–5 toxicity including 1.1% of patients developing symptomatic radionecrosis.

Salvage After SRS

- Zindler et al. (2014): Retrospective review of 443 patients with 1–3 brain metastases treated with RS alone. Salvage treatment for distant brain recurrence (DBR) in 25% of patients, 70% of which had ≤3 lesions. Actuarial DBR rates at 6, 12, and 24 months after primary SRS were 21, 41, and 54%, respectively. Median time to DBR: 5.6 months. DBR-RPA classes: I=WHO 0 or 1, ≥6 months from RS (OS 10 months); II = WHO 0 or 1, <6 months from RS (OS 5 months); III = WHO ≥2 (OS 3 months).
- Wake Forest (Farris et al. 2017): Retrospective evaluation of 737 patients treated with brain metastases with SRS alone, proposed metric of brain metastasis velocity (BMV) equal to the number of new brain metastases after SRS over time in years. Low-, intermediate-, and high-risk categories had significant difference in OS at 12.4 months (95% CI: 10.4–16.9), 8.2 months (95% CI, 5.0–9.7), and 4.3 months (95% CI: 2.6–6.7) respectively. Lower BMV was associated with decreased use of salvage WBRT ($p = 0.02$) and lower risk of neurological death (p = 0.008).

Meningioma

- Mayo Clinic (Stafford et al. 2001): Retrospective review of 190 consecutive patients with 206 meningiomas treated by SRS (median marginal dose 16 Gy; median target volume 8.2 cm^3). Prior surgery in 59% of patients; 12% of lesions with atypical or anaplastic histology; 77% of tumors involved the skull base. Five-year CSS for benign, atypical, and anaplastic tumors was 100, 76, and 0%, respectively; LC 93, 68, and 0%, respectively. Complications attributed to SRS in 13% of patients (CN deficits in 8%, symptomatic parenchymal changes in 3%, carotid artery stenosis in

1%, and cyst formation in 1%); decrease in functional status related to radiosurgery in six patients.

- University of Pittsburgh (Kondziolka et al. 1999a, b): Retrospective review of 99 consecutive patients treated with SRS (43%) or surgery followed by SRS (57%). Median marginal dose 16 Gy; median target volume 4.7 cm^3. Five patients previously treated with conventional RT; 89% of tumors adjacent to the skull base. At 10 years, 11% LF; PFS worse in patients with prior resections and multiple meningiomas. New or worsening neurologic symptoms in 5% of patients. By survey, 96% of patients considered treatment a success.

WHO Grade 1 Meningioma

- Germany (Fokas et al. 2014): Retrospective review of 318 patients with histologically confirmed (45%) or radiographically presumed (55%) benign meningioma treated with fractionated stereotactic RT (80%; median dose 55.8 Gy/31 fractions), hypofractionated stereotactic RT (15%; 40 Gy/10 fractions or 25–35 Gy/5–7 fractions), or SRS (5%) based on tumor size and proximity to critical structures. With median follow-up 50 months, 5- and 10-year LC, OS, and CSS were 93, 89, and 97%; and 88, 74, and 97%, respectively. On multivariate analysis, tumor location and age >66 years were significant predictors of LC and OS, respectively. Acute worsening of neurologic symptoms and/or clinically significant acute toxicity after RT in 2% of patients; no late grade ≥3 toxicity.
- University of Pittsburgh (Kondziolka et al. 2014): Retrospective review of 290 benign meningioma patients treated with GKRS (median marginal dose 15 Gy, median target volume 5.5 cm^3). Prior fractionated RT in 22 patients, STR in 126 patients, and recurrence after GTR in 22 patients. Overall tumor control 91%; 10- and 20-year actuarial PFS from the treated lesion were both 87%. Among symptomatic patients, 26%

improved, 54% remained stable, and 20% had a gradual worsening. No significant difference in control with prior craniotomy vs. primary GKRS; PFS worse in those with prior RT and higher-grade lesions.

■ Santacroce et al. (2012): Retrospective, multicenter review of 4565 consecutive patients with 5300 benign meningiomas treated with GKRS (median marginal dose 14 Gy; median target volume 4.8 cm^3). Results of 3768 lesions with >24 months follow-up reported. Tumor size decreased in 58% of cases, remained unchanged in 34%, and increased in 8%; overall control rate 92%. Five- and 10-year PFS 95 and 89%, respectively. Tumor control higher for presumed meningiomas vs. histologically confirmed grade I lesions, female vs. male patients, sporadic vs. multiple meningiomas, and skull base vs. convexity tumors. Permanent morbidity in 6.6%.

■ Prague (Kollová et al. 2007): Retrospective review of 400 benign meningiomas in 368 patients treated with SRS (median marginal dose 12.5 Gy; median target volume 4.4 cm^3). With median follow-up of 5 years, 70% of tumors decreased in size, 28% remained stable, and 2% increased in size. Actuarial LC 98%; worse in men and with <12 Gy. Temporary toxicity in 10% and permanent in 6%. Peritumoral edema worse with >16 Gy, age >60 years, no prior surgery, preexisting edema, tumor volume >10 cm^3, and anterior fossa location.

■ Mayo Clinic (Pollock et al. 2003): Retrospective review of 198 benign meningiomas <3.5 cm^3 in mean diameter treated surgically ($n = 136$) or with primary SRS ($n = 62$; mean marginal dose 18 Gy). No statistically significant difference in 3- and 7-year PFS for Simpson Grade I resections (100 and 96%, respectively) and SRS (100 and 95%, respectively). SRS associated with superior PFS relative to Simpson Grade ≥2 resections, and relative to surgery in general, fewer adjuvant treatments (3% vs. 15%) and fewer complications (10% vs. 22%).

- RTOG 0539 Low Risk (Rogers et al. 2020a, b): Phase II prospective cohort of observation after GTR or STR of a WHO grade 1 meningioma. Overall 60 patients eligible for analysis with 58 (93.4%) having undergone GTR, the 5-year and 10-year PFS were 89.4% and 85.0%. In patients with confirmed STR, 10-year PFS was 72.7%, with no incidence of grade 4 or 5 adverse events, reflecting the good outcomes for low-risk GTR meningioma but raise questions about management after STR.

WHO Grade 2 and 3 Meningioma

- Northwestern University (Kaur et al. 2014): Systematic review from 1994 to 2011 analyzing 21 English-language studies reporting tumor characteristics, treatment parameters, and clinical outcomes for atypical and malignant (anaplastic) meningiomas treated with adjuvant RT or SRS. Median 5-year PFS and OS for atypical lesions after adjuvant RT were 54 and 68%, respectively; anaplastic lesions: 48 and 56%, respectively. Outcomes data identified for only 23 patients treated with SRS (median marginal dose 18–19 Gy), generally with poor outcomes.
- UCSF (Kaprealian et al. 2016): Retrospective analysis of 280 patients with 438 meningioma. 5-year FFP for WHO grade 2 and 3 meningioma were 56% and 47%, respectively. Of WHO grade 3 meningiomas 87% failed within the prior SRS target volume, with 13% failing immediately adjacent to the volume. On MVA poorer FFP was associated with larger target volume and SRS after prior radiotherapy versus after prior surgery alone. No association was demonstrated between SRS dose and improved FFP for any grade meningioma.
- RTOG 0539 Intermediate Risk (Rogers et al. 2018): Phase II trial of conventionally fractionated RT (54 Gy in 30 Fx) for recurrent WHO grade 1 meningioma, and

WHO grade 2 meningioma with a GTR. Primary outcome 3-year PFS, actuarially 93.8% with no significant difference in PFS between participants with benign or atypical tumors ($p = 0.52$, HR 0.56), with no grade 3+ reported adverse events.

- RTOG 0539 High Risk (Rogers et al. 2018): Phase II trial of adjuvant radiation for recurrent atypical, STR atypical, or anaplastic meningioma. All participants received 60 Gy in 30 fractions, with large margins (1–2 cm) including extension beyond anatomic boundaries. Overall 57 patients enrolled with median follow-up of 4 years, with primary outcome being 3-year PFS at 58.8%, LC at 3-years was 68.9%, and OS was 78.6%. Overall, 1 patient (1.9%) experienced a late grade 5 AE due to radionecrosis. Adjuvant radiotherapy showed acceptable rates of toxicity with ongoing need for improvement in outcomes in this cohort of patients.

Skull Base

- NAGKC (Sheehan et al. 2014): Multi-institutional, retrospective review of 763 patients with sellar and/or parasellar meningiomas treated with GKRS (median marginal dose 13 Gy; median target volume 6.7 cm^3); 51% prior resection, and 4% prior RT. Median follow-up 67 months. Actuarial PFS at 5 and 10 years 95 and 82%, respectively; significant predictors of progression included >1 prior surgery, prior RT, and tumor marginal dose <13 Gy. Stability or improvement in neurologic symptoms in 86% of patients; CN V and VI improvement in 34% with preexisting deficits. Progression of existing neurologic symptoms in 14% of patients; new or worsening CN deficits in 10% (most likely CN V dysfunction). New or worsening endocrinopathy in 1.6% of patients.
- NAGKC (Starke et al. 2014): Multi-institution, retrospective review of 254 patients with

radiographically presumed (55%) or histologically confirmed (45%) benign petroclival meningioma treated with GKRS upfront (n = 140) or following surgery (114). Mean marginal dose 13.4 Gy; mean target volume 7.5 cm^3. With mean follow-up of 71 months, 9% of tumors increased in size, 52% remained stable, and 39% decreased; 94% of patients had stable or improved neurologic symptoms. PFS at 5 and 10 years was 93 and 84%, respectively. Multivariate predictors of favorable outcome included small tumor volume, female gender, no prior RT, and lower maximal dose.

- Park et al. (2014): Retrospective review of 74 patients with cerebellopontine angle (CPA) meningioma treated with GKRS; median marginal of dose 13 Gy, median target volume 3 cm^3. With median follow-up 40 months, 62% of tumors decreased in size, 35% remained stable, and 3% increased. PFS at 1 and 5 years was 98 and 95%, respectively. Neurological improvement in 31%, stability in 58%, and worsening of symptoms in 11% of patients (most likely trigeminal neuralgia); rate of improvement 1, 3, and 5 years after GKRS was 16, 31, and 40%, respectively. Asymptomatic peritumoral edema in 5% of patients; symptomatic adverse radiation effects in 9%.

Ongoing

- EORTC-1308/ROAM: Multicenter randomized controlled trial running in the United Kingdom evaluating the use of adjuvant radiation therapy versus observation in WHO grade II meningioma after GTR. Radiation therapy consists of 60 Gy in 30 fractions within 8–12 weeks of resection. Target accrual of 190 patients, currently enrolling.
- NRG-BN003: Multicenter randomized phase III trial evaluating observation versus adjuvant radiation

therapy after GTR of WHO grade II meningioma. Primary end point is PFS with radiation therapy consisting of 59.4 Gy in 33 fractions with target accrual of 148 patients, currently enrolling.

Acoustic Neuroma

- University of Pittsburgh (Lunsford et al. 2005): Retrospective review of GKRS outcomes for 829 vestibular schwannoma patients; median marginal dose 13 Gy, mean target volume 2.5 cm^3. Ten-year tumor control rate 97%; hearing preservation 77%. Toxicity notable for <1% facial neuropathy and <3% trigeminal symptoms.
- University of Pittsburg (Johnson et al. 2019): Retrospective review of long-term outcomes for 871 vestibular schwannoma patients, median follow-up 5.2 years (range 1–25). PFS 97% at 3 years, 95% at 5 years, and 94% at 10 years, with rates of serviceable hearing preservation of 68.4% at 5 years and 51.4% at 10 years. Overall 51 patients (5.8%) developed trigeminal neuropathy and 11 patients (1.3%) required surgical intervention for progression after SRS.

Surgery vs. SRS

- Marseille, France (Régis et al. 2002): Non-randomized, prospective series of GKRS ($n = 97$) vs. microsurgery ($n = 110$) for vestibular schwannoma with preoperative and postoperative questionnaire assessment. Median follow-up 4 years. GKRS universally superior in terms of facial motor function (0% vs. 37%), CN V disturbance (4% vs. 29%), hearing preservation (70% vs. 38%), overall functionality (91% vs. 61%), duration of hospitalization (3 vs. 23 days), and mean time missed from work (7 vs. 130 days).

Hypofractionated Stereotactic RT vs. SRS

- Amsterdam (Meijer et al. 2003): Prospective trial of single-fraction (n = 49) vs. fractionated linac-based SRS (n = 80) for acoustic neuroma; mean tumor diameter ~2.5 cm. Dentate patients treated with 20–25 Gy/5 fractions, and edentate patients treated with 10–12.5 Gy/1 fraction to the 80% isodose line. Median follow-up 33 months. Excellent tumor control (100% vs. 94%), preservation of hearing (75% vs. 61%), preservation of CN V (92% vs. 98%, statistically significant difference), and preservation of CN VII (93% vs. 97%) with both modalities.
- Japan (Morimoto et al. 2013): Retrospective review of 26 vestibular schwannomas treated with hypofractionated robotic radiosurgery to 18–25 Gy/3–5 fractions (median target volume 2.6 cm³). Progression defined as ≥2 mm 3D post-treatment tumor enlargement. Seven-year PFS and LC were 78 and 95%, respectively. Six reports of late grade ≥3 toxicity. Formal audiometric testing demonstrated 50% retention of pure tone averages.

Proton Beam Radiosurgery

- Harvard (Weber et al. 2003): Eighty-eight consecutive patients with vestibular schwannoma treated with 3 converging beams aligned to fiducial markers in the calvarium; maximum dose 13 Gy RBE, median target volume 1.4 cm³. Actuarial 5-year tumor control 94%, and preservation of CN's V and VII 89 and 91%, respectively, but serviceable hearing preservation 33%. Proton beam radiosurgery now only used for tumors <2 cm, and in patients without functional hearing.

Paraganglioma

- Pollock (2004): Retrospective, single-institution review of 42 patients with glomus jugulare tumors treated with single-session GKRS; mean marginal dose of 15 Gy, mean volume 13 cm^3. With median follow-up of 3.7 years, 31% decreased in size, 67% remained stable, and 2% progressed. Seven- and 10-year PFS were 100 and 75%, respectively. Hearing preservation 81% at 4 years, with 15% of patients developing new deficits including hearing loss, facial numbness, vocal cord paralysis, and vertigo.
- Mayo Clinic (Patel et al. 2018): Single-institution retrospective review of 85 patients treated from 1990 to 2017 with GKSRS with median follow-up of 66 months (range 7–202) and a median tumor volume of 11.6 cm^3. Five-year PFS was 98% with median marginal dose to the tumor of 16 Gy (range 12–18 Gy) in a single fraction. Overall, 1 (1%) patient required salvage with EBRT, and 2 (3%) patients experienced clinically worsening neuropathy resulting in vocal cord paralysis (CN X).

Hypofractionation

- Chun et al. (2014): Retrospective, single-institution review of 31 patients with skull base paragangliomas treated with robotic radiosurgery to a total dose of 25 Gy/5 fractions. With median follow-up 24 months, OS and LC were both 100%; tinnitus improved in 60% of patients. Overall tumor volume decreased by 37% (49% when analyzing subset of patients with ≥24-month follow-up). No grade ≥ 3 toxicity.

Surgery vs. SRS

- Gottfried et al. (2004): Meta-analysis of 7 surgical series (374 patients) and 8 GKRS series (142 patients) of glomus jugulare tumors; mean follow-up 4 and 3 years, respectively. LC 92% with surgery, 97% with GKRS. Complications notable for 8% morbidity from GKRS, 8% CSF leak from surgery, and 1.3% surgical mortality. Conclusion that both treatments are safe and efficacious, although inaccessibility of skull base limits selection of surgical candidates.

Pituitary Adenoma

- Sheehan et al. (2005a, b)): Systematic review of 35 peer-reviewed studies involving 1621 patients with pituitary adenoma treated with SRS. LC >90% achieved in most studies, with mean marginal dose ranging from 15 to 34 Gy/1 fraction. Weighted mean tumor control rate for all published studies 96%. Sixteen cases of damage to the optic apparatus with doses ranging from 0.7 to 12 Gy. Twenty-one new neuropathies from CN dysfunction, nearly half of which were transient. Risks of hypopituitarism, RT-induced neoplasia, and cerebral vasculopathy lower with SRS than historical rates with fractionated RT. Heterogeneous quantification of endocrinological remission for Cushing disease, acromegaly, prolactinoma, and Nelson syndrome, with wide variation of endocrine control. Hormone improvement anywhere from 3 months to 8 years after SRS, although levels typically normalize within 2 years.

Hypofractionation

- Iwata et al. (2011): Single-institution retrospective review of 100 patients with recurrent/residual nonfunctioning pituitary adenomas without a history of prior RT treated with SRS to 21–25 Gy/3–5 fractions; median target volume 5.1 cm^3. Three-year OS and LC both 98%. One case of visual disturbance after treatment, three cases of hypopituitarism in patients not previously on hormone replacement therapy, and three cases of transient cyst enlargement.

Hormone Control and Risk of Hypopituitarism

- Xu et al. (2013): Retrospective, single-institution review of 262 pituitary adenoma patients treated by SRS with thorough endocrine assessments immediately before treatment, and then again at regular follow-up intervals. Tumor control 89% and remission of endocrine abnormalities in 72% of functional adenoma patients. Thirty percent rate of new hypopituitarism; increased risk with suprasellar extension and higher marginal dose, but not with tumor volume, prior surgery, prior RT, or age at SRS.
- Mayo Clinic (Graffeo et al. 2018): Retrospective review of 97 patients with pituitary adenoma undergoing single-fraction SRS with at least 24 months of endocrine follow-up. Overall median follow-up of 48 months (IQR 34–68) with 27 (28%) patients developing pituitary insufficiency at a median of 22 months. Hypopituitarism with a mean gland dose of <11.0 Gy was 5% (95% CI 0–11%) at 5 years and for a mean gland dose of ≥11.0 Gy was 51% (95% CI 34–65%) at 5 years. Pituitary dysfunction increases in a time and dose-dependent manner after SRS for pituitary adenoma.

Vascular Malformations

Arteriovenous Malformation (AVM)

- Tokyo, Japan (Maruyama et al. 2005): Retrospective, single-institution review of 500 AVM patients status post-definitive treatment with GKRS (mean dose 21 Gy; median Spetzler-Martin grade III). Pre-GKRS rate of spontaneous hemorrhage ~6%; cumulative 4-year obliteration rate 81%, 5-year rate 91%. Hemorrhage risk reduced by 54% during the latency period post-GKRS/pre-obliteration, and 88% after obliteration; greatest risk reduction in those who initially presented with hemorrhage.
- University of Maryland (Koltz et al. 2013): Retrospective review of 102 patients treated with single-fraction or staged SRS for AVM's stratified by Spetzler-Martin grade. With mean follow-up of 8.5 years, overall nidus obliteration was 75% with 19% morbidity, both of which correlated with Spetzler-Martin grade. For Grade I–V lesions, obliteration achieved in 100, 89, 86, 54, and 0% of cases. For AVMs that were not completely obliterated, the mean reduction in nidus volume was 69%.
- University of Virginia (Ding et al. 2014): Retrospective review of 398 Spetzler-Martin grade III AVMs treated with SRS (median target volume 2.8 cm^3, median prescription 20 Gy). With median 68 months clinical follow-up, complete obliteration in 69% of lesions after median of 46 months from SRS. Significant predictors of response included prior hemorrhage, size <3 cm, deep venous drainage, and eloquent location. Annual risk for hemorrhage during the latency period was 1.7%. Symptomatic radiation-induced complications in 12% of patients (permanent in 4%); independent predictors included absence of pre-SRS rupture and presence of a single draining vein.

Conclusion: SRS for Spetzler-Martin grade III lesions is comparable to surgery in long term.

- Harvard (Hattangadi-Gluth et al. 2014): Retrospective review of 248 consecutive patients with 254 cerebral AVMs treated with single-fraction proton beam stereotactic radiosurgery; median target volume 3.5 cm^3, 23% in eloquent/deep locations, and median prescription dose 15 Gy RBE. With median 35 months follow-up, 65% obliteration rate, median time to obliteration 31 months; 5- and 10-year cumulative incidence of total obliteration was 70 and 91%, respectively. Univariate and multivariate analyses showed location and smaller target volume to be independent predictors of total obliteration; smaller volume and higher prescription dose also significant on univariate analysis.

- Harvard (Barker et al. 2003): Retrospective review of toxicity data in 1250 AVM patients treated with stereotactic proton beam radiosurgery. Median follow-up 6.5 years, median dose 10.5 Gy, median target volume 33.7 cm^3 (23% <10 cm^3). Permanent radiation-related deficits in 4% of patients; median time to complications 1.1 years. Complication rate related to dose, volume, deep location, and age; rate <0.5% with <12 Gy.

- Nagasaki, Japan (Matsuo et al. 2014): Median 15.6-year results of 51 AVM patients treated with linear accelerator-based radiosurgery; median prescription 15 Gy, median target volume 4.5 cm^3, median Spetzler-Martin grade II. Actuarial obliteration rates after 5 and 15 years were 54 and 68%, which increased to 61 and 90% when allowing for salvage treatments. Obliteration rate significantly related to target volume ≥4 cm^3, marginal dose ≥12 Gy, and Spetzler-Martin grade I (vs. others) on univariate analysis (target volume also significant on multivariate analysis). Post-treatment hemorrhage observed in 7 cases (14%), predominantly within latency period; actuarial posttreatment bleeding rate ~5% during the first 2 years, and 1.1% upon final observation. Actuarial symptomatic radiation injury rates at 5 and 15 years were 12 and 19%, respectively; target volume ≥ 4 cm^3 and location (lobular vs. other) were significantly associated with radiation injury on univariate and multivariate analysis. Cyst formation in five cases (9.8% of patients; three asymptomatic, two treated with resection, and one resolved with steroids).

Staged AVM Treatment

- Yamamoto et al. (2012): Thirty-one patients retrospectively identified who underwent intentional 2-stage GKRS for 32 AVMs with nidus >10 cm^3 (mean target volume 16 cm^3, maximum 56 cm^3). Low radiation doses (12–16 Gy) given to the lesion periphery during the first treatment; second session planned 36 months after the first. Complete nidus obliteration in 65% of patients, and marked shrinkage in the remaining 35%. Mild symptomatic GKRS-related complications in 2 patients.
- Ding et al. (2013): Eleven patients with large AVMs (31 ± 19 cm^3) divided into 3–7 cm^3 sub-targets for sequential treatment by robotic radiosurgery at 1–4-week intervals. Forward and inverse planning used to optimize 95% coverage for delivery of 16–20 Gy; mean conformality index 0.65.

AVM Treatment Versus Medical Management

- ARUBA Trial (Mohr et al. 2020): Prospective randomized control trial of medical management versus neurologic intervention (surgery or radiosurgery) for unruptured AVM. Overall 226 patients randomized with cessation at interim analysis due to futility. Primary outcome was death from any cause or symptomatic stroke, long-term results with 50.4 months follow-up showed 3.4 events per 100 patient in years in the medical management arm versus 12.3 per 100 patients years in the intervention arm (HR 0.31; 95% CI 0.17–0.56). Primary critique of this trial is the short follow-up time at cessation of accrual and the number of early events in the intervention arm.

Cavernous Malformation

- Poorthuis et al. (2014): Systematic review and meta-regression analysis of 63 cohorts involving 3424 patients. Composite outcome of death, nonfatal intracranial hemorrhage, or new/worse persistent focal neurological deficit was 6.6 per 100 person-years after surgical excision ($n = 2684$), and 5.4 after SRS ($n = 740$; median dose 16 Gy). However, lesions treated with SRS significantly smaller than those treated surgically (14 mm vs. 19 mm).
- University of Pittsburgh (Hasegawa et al. 2002a, b): Retrospective review of 82 consecutive patients treated with SRS for hemorrhagic cavernous malformations; annual hemorrhage rate 34%, excluding the first hemorrhage. Mean marginal dose 16.2 Gy, mean volume 1.85 cm^3. With mean follow-up of 5 years, average hemorrhage rate for the first 2 years after radiosurgery was 12%, followed by <1% from years 2 through 12. Eleven patients (13%) had new neurological symptoms without hemorrhage after radiosurgery.

Trigeminal Neuralgia

Primary Treatment

- Marseille, France (Régis et al. 2006): Phase I prospective trial of GKRS (median dose 85 Gy) in 100 patients with trigeminal neuralgia; 42% with history of prior surgery. At 12 months, 83% pain free, 58% pain free and off medication; salvage rate 17%. Side effects included mild facial paresthesia in 6% and hyperesthesia in 4%.
- University of Virginia (Sheehan et al. 2005a, b): GKRS used to treat trigeminal neuralgia in 151 consecutive patients with median 19 months follow-up. Median time to pain relief was 24 days; at 3 years, 34% of patients were pain free, and 70% of patients had improvement in pain. Twelve patients experienced new onset of facial numbness after treatment, which correlated with repeat GKRS. Right-sided neuralgia and prior neurectomy correlated with pain-free outcomes on univariate analysis; multivariate analysis similarly significant for right-sided neuralgia.
- Brussels, Belgium and Marseilles, France (Massager et al. 2007): Retrospective stratification of 358 trigeminal neuralgia patients into 3 dosimetric groups: <90 Gy (no blocking), 90 Gy (no blocking), and 90 Gy with blocking. Excellent pain control in 66% vs. 77% vs. 84%; good pain control in 81%, 85%, and 90%. Mild trigeminal toxicity in 15% vs. 21% vs. 49%; bothersome toxicity in 1.4% vs. 2.4% vs. 10%.
- Brisman (2007): Review of 85 patients with trigeminal neuralgia treated with microvascular decompression (MVD, n = 24) or GKRS (n = 61) and followed prospectively. Complete pain relief at 12 and 18 months achieved in 68% of MVD patients, and 58 and 24% of GKRS patients; partial pain relief more equivalent. No permanent complications.

- Tuleasca et al. (2018): Systematic review including 65 retrospective and prospective studies of 6461 patients treated with radiosurgery (GK, linac, CK) for trigeminal neuralgia. Maximal doses were 60–97 Gy for GK, 50–90 Gy for linac, and 66–90 Gy for CK within this series of studies. Actuarial pain relief was a median of 52.1% (range 28.6–100%), with median rate of recurrence of 23% (range 0–52.2%).

Retreatment

- UCSF (Sanchez-Mejia et al. 2005): Retrospective review of 32 patients retreated for trigeminal neuralgia with MVD (n = 19), radiofrequency ablation (RFA, n = 5), or SRS (n = 8) from an initial cohort of 209 patients. Retreatment rate with RFA (42%) significantly greater than the rate of retreatment with either MVD (20%) or SRS (8%).
- Columbia (Brisman 2003): Retrospective review of 335 patients with primary trigeminal neuralgia treated to a maximum dose of 75 Gy by GKRS, and then 45 retreated to a maximum dose of 40 Gy GKRS (mean interval 18 months). Final pain relief was 50% or greater in 62% of patients; absence of prior surgery was an independent predictor of response to retreatment. Significant dysesthesias in 2 patients; no other serious complications.
- Zhang et al. (2005): Retrospective study of 40 trigeminal neuralgia patients initially treated with 75 Gy GKRS, and then retreated with 40 Gy GKRS. Landmark-based registration algorithm used to determine spatial relationship between primary and retreatment isocenters. Trend toward better pain relief with farther distance between isocenters; however, neither placing the second isocenter proximal or distal to the brainstem was significant. Mean distance 2.9 mm

in complete or nearly complete responders vs. 1.9 mm in all others.

- Dvorak et al. (2009): Retrospective study of 28 trigeminal neuralgia patients initially treated to median 80 Gy GKRS, then retreated to median 45 Gy GKRS after a median 18-month interval. Univariate analysis showed no significant predictors of pain control or complication. However, when combining peer-reviewed retreatment series (215 total patients), both improved pain control and new trigeminal dysfunction were associated with greater dose: cumulative dose >130 Gy likely to result in >50% pain control as well as >20% risk of new dysfunction.
- University of Pittsburgh (Park et al. 2014): Retrospective review of a single institution to evaluate outcomes after repeat GK radiosurgery for trigeminal neuralgia. Overall 119 patients identified with median interval of 26 months between initial and repeat GKSRS, and median maximal target dose at retreatment was 70 Gy (range 50–90 Gy). Overall 87% of patients received initial pain relief (BNI score I-IIIb), with 44.2% having continued relief after 5 years. Sensory deficits occurred in 25 (21%) of patients between 2 and 18 months, with 76% being classified as mild or not bothersome.

Pineal Tumors

- University of Pittsburgh (Hasegawa et al. 2002a, b): Retrospective review of 16 patients treated with SRS for pineal parenchymal tumors (10 pineocytomas, 2 mixed pineocytoma/pineoblastoma, and 4 pineoblastoma). Mean dose 15 Gy, mean target volume 5 cm^3. Actuarial 2 and 5 year OS 75 and 67%, respectively; CR 29%, PR 57%, SD 14%. LC 100%

although 4 patients died from leptomeningeal or extracranial spread. Two cases of gaze palsy 7 and 13 months after SRS attributed to treatment, one resolved with steroids and the other persisted until death.

- Marseille, France (Reyns et al. 2006): Retrospective review of 13 patients with pineal parenchymal tumors (8 pineocytomas and 5 pineoblastomas) treated with SRS (mean marginal dose 15 Gy). With mean follow-up 34 months, LC 100%; 2 pineoblastomas progressed outside of SRS field resulting in death. No major mortality or morbidity related to SRS.

- United Kingdom (Yianni et al. 2012): Retrospective review of 44 patients with pineal tumors treated with SRS (11 pineal parenchymal tumors, 6 astrocytomas, 3 ependymomas, 2 papillary epithelial tumors, and 2 germ cell tumors). Mean dose 18.2 Gy, mean target volume 3.8 cm^3. One- and 5-year PFS 93 and 77%, respectively, but separating aggressive tumors from indolent lesions showed 5-year PFS 47 and 91%, respectively. Tumor grade, prior RT, and radionecrosis associated with worse outcome.

Functional Disorders

Epilepsy

- UCSF (Chang et al. 2010): Prospective, randomized trial involving 30 patients with intractable medial temporal lobe epilepsy treated with 20 Gy/1 fraction vs. 24 Gy/1 by GKRS to the amygdala, 2 cm of the anterior hippocampus, and parahippocampal gyrus. Nonsignificant difference in seizure control between arms (59% vs. 77%), although early MRI alterations predictive of long-term seizure remission.

Parkinson Disease and Essential Tremor

- Japan (Ohye et al. 2012): Prospective, multicenter study of 72 patients with intractable Parkinson disease or essential tremor treated with selective thalamotomy by GKRS with a single 130 Gy shot to the lateral part of the ventralis intermedius nucleus (located 45% of the thalamic length from the anterior tip). Excellent or good response with improved tremor in 43 of 53 patients (81%) who completed 24 months of follow-up. No permanent clinical complications.
- University of Pittsburgh (Kondziolka et al. 2008): Retrospective review of GKRS thalamotomy in 31 patients with medically refractory essential tremor. Nucleus ventralis intermedius treated with 130–140 Gy in a single fraction. With median follow-up of 26 months, mean tremor score improved by 54%, and mean handwriting score improved by 39%, with the majority of patients (69%) seeing improvement in both. Permanent mild right hemiparesis and speech impairment in 1 patient 6 months after radiosurgery; 1 patient with transient right hemiparesis and dysphagia.
- Martinez-Moreno et al. (2018): Systematic review of 34 studies on SRS for tremor, 3 prospective studies and 31 retrospective studies. SRS thalamotomy to a dose of 130–150 Gy in a single fraction resulted in mean rate of tremor reduction of 88% with a mean complication rate of 17%. Most studies limited by lack of long-term follow-up; however, treatments were effective and well tolerated and recommended as a treatment option by the ISRS.

References

Andrews DW, et al. Whole brain radiation therapy with or without stereotactic radiosurgery boost for patients with one to three brain metastases: phase III results of the RTOG 9508 randomised trial. Lancet. 2004;363:1665–72.

Aoyama H, et al. Stereotactic radiosurgery plus whole-brain radiation therapy vs. stereotactic radiosurgery alone for treatment of brain metastases: a randomized controlled trial. JAMA. 2006;295:2483–91.

Barker FG, et al. Dose-volume prediction of radiation-related complications after proton beam radiosurgery for cerebral arteriovenous malformations. J Neurosurg. 2003;99:254–63.

Bhatnagar AK, Flickinger JC, Kondziolka D, Lunsford LD. Stereotactic radiosurgery for four or more intracranial metastases. Radiat Oncol Biol. 2006;64:898–903.

Brisman R. Repeat gamma knife radiosurgery for trigeminal neuralgia. Stereotact Funct Neurosurg. 2003;81:43–9.

Brisman R. Microvascular decompression vs. gamma knife radiosurgery for typical trigeminal neuralgia: preliminary findings. Stereotact Funct Neurosurg. 2007;85:94–8.

Brown PD, et al. Effect of radiosurgery alone versus radiosurgery with whole brain radiation therapy on cognitive function in patients with 1 to 3 brain metastases: a randomized clinical trial. JAMA. 2016;316(4):401–9.

Brown PD, et al. Postoperative stereotactic radiosurgery compared with whole brain radiotherapy for resected metastatic brain disease (NCCTG N107C/CEC.3): a multicentre randomised controlled, phase 3 trial. Lancet Oncol. 2017;18(8):1049–60.

Chang EL, et al. Neurocognition in patients with brain metastases treated with radiosurgery or radiosurgery plus whole-brain irradiation: a randomised controlled trial. Lancet Oncol. 2009;10:1037–44.

Chang EF, et al. Predictors of efficacy after stereotactic radiosurgery for medial temporal lobe epilepsy. Neurology. 2010;74:165–72.

Chen WC, et al. Efficacy and safety of Stereotactic radiosurgery for brainstem metastases: a systematic review and meta-analysis. JAMA Oncol. 2021;7(7):1–9.

Chun SG, et al. A retrospective analysis of tumor volumetric responses to five-fraction stereotactic radiotherapy for paragangliomas of the head and neck (glomus tumors). Stereotact Funct Neurosurg. 2014;92:153–9.

Ding C, et al. Multi-staged robotic stereotactic radiosurgery for large cerebral arteriovenous malformations. Radiother Oncol. 2013;109:452–6.

Ding D, et al. Radiosurgery for Spetzler-Martin Grade III arteriovenous malformations. J Neurosurg. 2014;120:959–69.

Donnet A, Tamura M, Valade D, Régis J. Trigeminal nerve radiosurgical treatment in intractable chronic cluster headache: unexpected high toxicity. Neurosurgery. 2006;59:1252–7. discussion 1257

Dvorak T, et al. Retreatment of trigeminal neuralgia with Gamma Knife radiosurgery: is there an appropriate cumulative dose? Clinical article. J Neurosurg. 2009;111:359–64.

Farris M, et al. Brain metastasis velocity: a novel prognostic metric predictive of overall survival and freedom from whole-brain radiation therapy after distant brain failure following upfront radiosurgery alone. Int J Radiat Oncol Biol Phys. 2017;98(1):131–41.

Fokas E, Henzel M, Surber G, Hamm K, Engenhart-Cabillic R. Stereotactic radiation therapy for benign meningioma: long-term outcome in 318 patients. Int J Radiat Oncol Biol Phys. 2014;89:569–75.

Gaspar L, et al. Recursive partitioning analysis (RPA) of prognostic factors in three Radiation Therapy Oncology Group (RTOG) brain metastases trials. Radiat Oncol Biol. 1997;37:745–51.

Gottfried ON, Liu JK, Couldwell WT. Comparison of radiosurgery and conventional surgery for the treatment of glomus jugulare tumors. Neurosurg Focus. 2004;17:E4.

Graffeo CS, et al. Hypopituitarism after single-fraction pituitary adenoma radiosurgery: dosimetric analysis based on patients treated using contemporary techniques. Int J Radiat Oncol Biol Phys. 2018;101(3):618–23.

Hasegawa T, Kondziolka D, Hadjipanayis CG, Flickinger JC, Lunsford LD. The role of radiosurgery for the treatment of pineal parenchymal tumors. Neurosurgery. 2002a;51:880–9.

Hasegawa T, et al. Long-term results after stereotactic radiosurgery for patients with cavernous malformations. Neurosurgery. 2002b;50:1190–7; discussion 1197–8.

Hattangadi-Gluth JA, et al. Single-fraction proton beam stereotactic radiosurgery for cerebral arteriovenous malformations. Int J Radiat Oncol Biol Phys. 2014;89:338–46.

https://academic.oup.com/jjco/article/43/8/805/895136.

Iwata H, et al. Hypofractionated stereotactic radiotherapy with CyberKnife for nonfunctioning pituitary adenoma: high local control with low toxicity. Neuro-Oncology. 2011;13:916–22.

Johnson S, et al. Long term results of primary radiosurgery for vestibular schawannomas. J Neuro-Oncol. 2019;145:247–55.

Kano H, et al. Stereotactic radiosurgery for intractable cluster headache: an initial report from the North American Gamma Knife Consortium. J Neurosurg. 2011;114:1736–43.

Kaprealian T, et al. Parameters influencing local control of meningiomas treated with radiosurgery. J Neuro-oncol. 2016;128:357–64.

Kaur G, et al. Adjuvant radiotherapy for atypical and malignant meningiomas: a systematic review. Neuro-Oncology. 2014;16:628–36.

Kocher M, et al. Linac radiosurgery versus whole brain radiotherapy for brain metastases. A survival comparison based on the RTOG recursive partitioning analysis. Strahlenther Onkol. 2004;180:263–7.

Kocher M, et al. Adjuvant whole-brain radiotherapy versus observation after radiosurgery or surgical resection of one to three cerebral metastases: results of the EORTC 22952-26001 study. J Clin Oncol. 2011;29:134–41.

Kollová A, et al. Gamma Knife surgery for benign meningioma. J Neurosurg. 2007;107:325–36.

Koltz MT, et al. Long-term outcome of Gamma Knife stereotactic radiosurgery for arteriovenous malformations graded by the Spetzler-Martin classification. J Neurosurg. 2013;118:74–83.

Kondziolka D, Patel A, Lunsford LD, Kassam A, Flickinger JC. Stereotactic radiosurgery plus whole brain radiotherapy versus radiotherapy alone for patients with multiple brain metastases. Radiat Oncol Biol. 1999a;45:427–34.

Kondziolka D, Levy EI, Niranjan A, Flickinger JC, Lunsford LD. Long-term outcomes after meningioma radiosurgery: physician and patient perspectives. J Neurosurg. 1999b;91:44–50.

Kondziolka D, et al. Gamma knife thalamotomy for essential tremor. J Neurosurg. 2008;108:111–7.

Kondziolka D, Patel AD, Kano H, Flickinger JC, Lunsford LD. Long-term outcomes after gamma knife radiosurgery for meningiomas. Am J Clin Oncol. 2014;39(5):453–7. https://doi.org/10.1097/COC.0000000000000080.

Lad SP, et al. Cyberknife targeting the pterygopalatine ganglion for the treatment of chronic cluster headaches. Neurosurgery. 2007;60:E580–1; discussion E581.

Linskey ME, et al. The role of stereotactic radiosurgery in the management of patients with newly diagnosed brain metastases: a systematic review and evidence-based clinical practice guideline. J Neuro-Oncol. 2010;96:45–68.

Lunsford LD, Niranjan A, Flickinger JC, Maitz A, Kondziolka D. Radiosurgery of vestibular schwannomas: summary of experience in 829 cases. J Neurosurg. 2005;102(Suppl):195–9.

Mahajan A, et al. Post-operative stereotactic radiosurgery versus observation for completely resected brain metastases: a single-centre, randomised, controlled, phase 3 trial. Lancet Oncol. 2017;18(8):1040–8.

Martinez-Moreno NE, et al. Stereotactic radiosurgery for tremor: systemic review. J Neurosurg. 2018;1:1–12.

Maruyama K, et al. The risk of hemorrhage after radiosurgery for cerebral arteriovenous malformations. N Engl J Med. 2005;352:146–53.

Massager N, et al. Influence of nerve radiation dose in the incidence of trigeminal dysfunction after trigeminal neuralgia radiosurgery. Neurosurgery. 2007;60:681–7; discussion 687–8.

Matsuo T, Kamada K, Izumo T, Hayashi N, Nagata I. Linear accelerator-based radiosurgery alone for arteriovenous malformation: more than 12 years of observation. Int J Radiat Oncol Biol Phys. 2014;89:576–83.

McClelland S, Tendulkar RD, Barnett GH, Neyman G, Suh JH. Long-term results of radiosurgery for refractory cluster headache. Neurosurgery. 2006;59:1258–62; discussion 1262–3.

Meijer OWM, Vandertop WP, Baayen JC, Slotman BJ. Single-fraction vs. fractionated linac-based stereotactic radiosurgery for vestibular schwannoma: a single-institution study. Radiat Oncol Biol. 2003;56:1390–6.

Mohr JP, et al. Medical management with interventional therapy versus medical management alone for unruptured brain arteriovenous malformations (ARUBA): final follow-up of a multicenter, non-blinded, randomised controlled trial. Lancet Neurol. 2020;19(7):573–81.

Ohye C, et al. Gamma knife thalamotomy for Parkinson disease and essential tremor: a prospective multicenter study. Neurosurgery. 2012;70:526–35; discussion 535–6.

Park S-H, Kano H, Niranjan A, Flickinger JC, Lunsford LD. Stereotactic radiosurgery for cerebellopontine angle meningiomas. J Neurosurg. 2014;120:708–15.

Patel NS, et al. Long-term tumor control following stereotactic radiosurgery for jugular paraganglioma using 3D volumetric segmentation. J Neurosurg. 2018;1:1–9.

Pollock BE. Stereotactic radiosurgery in patients with glomus jugulare tumors. Neurosurg Focus. 2004;17:E10.

Pollock BE, Kondziolka D. Stereotactic radiosurgical treatment of sphenopalatine neuralgia. Case report. J Neurosurg. 1997;87:450–3.

Pollock BE, Stafford SL, Utter A, Giannini C, Schreiner SA. Stereotactic radiosurgery provides equivalent tumor control to Simpson Grade 1 resection for patients with small- to medium-size meningiomas. Radiat Oncol Biol. 2003;55:1000–5.

Poorthuis MH, Klijn CJ, Algra A, Rinkel GJ, Al-Shahi Salman R. Treatment of cerebral cavernous malformations: a systematic review and meta-regression analysis. J Neurol Neurosurg Psychiatry. 2014;85(12):1319–23.

Régis J, et al. Functional outcome after gamma knife surgery or microsurgery for vestibular schwannomas. J Neurosurg. 2002;97:1091–100.

Régis J, et al. Prospective controlled trial of gamma knife surgery for essential trigeminal neuralgia. J Neurosurg. 2006;104:913–24.

Reyns N, et al. The role of Gamma Knife radiosurgery in the treatment of pineal parenchymal tumours. Acta Neurochir. 2006;148:5–11; discussion 11.

Rogers CL, et al. Intermediate-risk meningioma: initial outcomes from NRG Oncology RTOG 0539. J Neurosurg. 2018;129(1):35–47.

Rogers CL, et al. Low-risk meningioma: outcomes from NRG-Oncology/RTOG 0539. Neuro-Oncology. 2020a;22(Supplement_2):ii55–6.

Rogers CL, et al. High-risk meningioma: initial outcomes from NRG Oncology/RTOG 0539. Int J Radiat Oncol Biol Phys. 2020b;106(4):790–9.

Sanchez-Mejia RO, et al. Recurrent or refractory trigeminal neuralgia after microvascular decompression, radiofrequency ablation, or radiosurgery. Neurosurg Focus. 2005;18:e12.

Santacroce A, et al. Long-term tumor control of benign intracranial meningiomas after radiosurgery in a series of 4565 patients. Neurosurgery. 2012;70:32–9; discussion 39.

Shaw E, et al. Single dose radiosurgical treatment of recurrent previously irradiated primary brain tumors and brain metastases: final report of RTOG protocol 90-05. Radiat Oncol Biol. 2000;47:291–8.

Sheehan J, Pan H-C, Stroila M, Steiner L. Gamma knife surgery for trigeminal neuralgia: outcomes and prognostic factors. J Neurosurg. 2005a;102:434–41.

Sheehan JP, et al. Stereotactic radiosurgery for pituitary adenomas: an intermediate review of its safety, efficacy, and role in the neurosurgical treatment armamentarium. J Neurosurg. 2005b;102:678–91.

Sheehan JP, et al. Gamma Knife radiosurgery for sellar and parasellar meningiomas: a multicenter study. J Neurosurg. 2014;120:1268–77.

Sneed PK, et al. Radiosurgery for brain metastases: is whole brain radiotherapy necessary? Radiat Oncol Biol. 1999;43:549–58.

Sneed PK, et al. A multi-institutional review of radiosurgery alone vs. radiosurgery with whole brain radiotherapy as the initial management of brain metastases. Radiat Oncol Biol. 2002;53:519–26.

Soliman H, et al. Consensus Contouring Guidelines for Postoperative Completely Resected Cavity Stereotactic Radiosurgery for Brain Metastases. Int J Radiat Oncol Biol Phys. 2018;100(2):436–42.

Soltys SG, et al. Stereotactic radiosurgery of the postoperative resection cavity for brain metastases. Radiat Oncol Biol. 2008;70:187–93.

Stafford SL, et al. Meningioma radiosurgery: tumor control, outcomes, and complications among 190 consecutive patients. Neurosurgery. 2001;49:1029–37; discussion 1037–8.

Starke R, et al. Stereotactic radiosurgery of petroclival meningiomas: a multicenter study. J Neuro-Oncol. 2014;119(1):169–76. https://doi.org/10.1007/s11060-014-1470-x.

Tuleasca C, et al. Stereotactic radiosurgery for trigeminal neuralgia: a systematic review. J Neurosurg. 2018;130(3):733–57.

Weber DC, et al. Proton beam radiosurgery for vestibular schwannoma: tumor control and cranial nerve toxicity. Neurosurgery. 2003;53:577–86; discussion 586–8.

Xu Z, Lee Vance M, Schlesinger D, Sheehan JP. Hypopituitarism after stereotactic radiosurgery for pituitary adenomas. Neurosurgery. 2013;72(630–7):636–7.

Yamamoto M, et al. Long-term follow-up results of intentional 2-stage Gamma Knife surgery with an interval of at least 3 years for arteriovenous malformations larger than 10 cm^3. J Neurosurg. 2012;117(Suppl):126–34.

Yamamoto M, et al. Stereotactic radiosurgery for patients with multiple brain metastases (JLGK0901): a multi-institutional prospective observational study. Lancet Oncol. 2014;15(4):387–95.

Yianni J, et al. Stereotactic radiosurgery for pineal tumours. Br J Neurosurg. 2012;26:361–6.

Zhang P, Brisman R, Choi J, Li X. Where to locate the isocenter? The treatment strategy for repeat trigeminal neuralgia radiosurgery. Radiat Oncol Biol. 2005;62:38–43.

Zindler JD, Slotman BJ, Lagerwaard FJ. Patterns of distant brain recurrences after radiosurgery alone for newly diagnosed brain metastases: implications for salvage therapy. Radiother Oncol. 2014;112(2):212–6.

Chapter 4
Spine

**Jessica Chew, Matthew S. Susko, David R. Raleigh,
Igor J. Barani, David A. Larson, and Steve E. Braunstein**

Pearls

- The spinal cord begins at the foramen magnum and, in
  adults, typically ends at the level of L1–L2. Below the
  termination of the cord, the spinal subarachnoid space

J. Chew (✉) · M. S. Susko · S. E. Braunstein
Department of Radiation Oncology, University of California, San
Francisco, San Francisco, CA, USA
e-mail: Jessica.Chew@ucsf.edu; Matthew.Susko@ucsf.edu;
steve.braunstein@ucsf.edu

D. R. Raleigh
Departments of Radiation Oncology and Neurological Surgery,
University of California, San Francisco, San Francisco, CA, USA
e-mail: david.raleigh@ucsf.edu

I. J. Barani
Department of Radiation Oncology, Barrow Neurological Institute,
Phoenix, AZ, USA

D. A. Larson
(deceased), Departments of Radiation Oncology and Neurological
Surgery, University of California, San Francisco, San Francisco, CA,
USA
e-mail: david.larson@ucsf.edu

© The Author(s), under exclusive license to Springer Nature   89
Switzerland AG 2023
R. A. Sethi et al. (eds.), *Handbook of Evidence-Based
Stereotactic Radiosurgery and Stereotactic Body Radiotherapy*,
https://doi.org/10.1007/978-3-031-33156-5_4

extends to S2–S3, and the spinal canal continues inferiorly into the coccyx.

- Metastases to the vertebrae and epidural space compose the vast majority of tumors adjacent to the spinal cord (Linstadt and Nakamura 2010) and are the most common SBRT treatment indication.
- Primary spinal cord tumors, such as chordoma and chondrosarcoma, account for 4–6% of all CNS neoplasms and are slightly more common in pediatric patients.
- Primary tumors involving the spinal cord typically originate within the spinal canal (65%) but may also arise from the spinal cord (10%) or vertebral bodies (10%).
- Presentation ranges from incidental discovery on surveillance imaging (especially in patients on high-dose steroids) to full paralysis, but the most common complaint is pain.
- Brown-Séquard syndrome: Ipsilateral motor and fine touch impairment, and contralateral loss of pain and temperature sensation.
- Crude local control (LC) after spine SBRT for spine metastases ranges from 70 to 100% (Lo et al. 2010; Sciubba et al. 2021); LC with conventional radiotherapy is approximately 86% for non-mass-type metastases, but falls to 46% for bulky lesions (Mizumoto et al. 2011).
- The risk–benefit ratio for SBRT treatment of meningioma, schwannoma, and malignant tumors of the spinal cord (glioblastoma, ependymoma, and metastases) relative to standard fractionation is not known.
- SBRT should be performed before cement kyphoplasty to prevent extravasation of active tumor into the epidural space (Cruz et al. 2014; Lis et al. 2018); however, kyphoplasty prior to SBRT may be safe for patients without epidural spinal cord compression (Barzilai et al. 2018).

Treatment indications

ASTRO 2017 guidelines for general spine SBRT (Lutz et al. 2017)	■ Previously radiated location(s) ■ Required relative sparing of adjacent neural structures ■ Favor enrollment on a clinical trial or registry
ISRS guidelines for spine SBRT outside clinical trial (Husain et al. 2017)	■ Oligometastatic spine disease ■ Radioresistant histology (e.g., renal cell carcinoma, melanoma, sarcoma) ■ Paraspinal extension contiguous to spine
Spinal cord compression	■ Limited compression (1–2 segments) ■ Subacute presentation (outcome unlikely to be impacted by protracted SBRT planning) ■ Re-irradiation ■ Postoperative after separation surgery for radioresistant primary
Primary spinal cord neoplasms	■ Postoperative adjuvant setting ■ Salvage

Workup

- H&P with emphasis on neurologic components.
- Review of systems, including:
    - Focal weakness.
    - Focal sensory changes.
    - Bowel or bladder incontinence, and perianal numbness which could indicate cauda equina involvement.
    - Back pain.

- Laboratories not typically required, except in cases where adjacent viscera may be invaded or if there is concern for hematologic malignancy (then CBC, CMP, LFTs, etc.).
- Imaging.
  - MRI spine with gadolinium remains the gold standard for assessment of spinal cord neoplasms and is also critical for SBRT targeting.
  - CT myelogram (standard or metrizamide enhanced) is often useful in patients with metallic vertebral implants or a permanent pacemaker. At some institutions, CT myelograms are standard practice for spine SBRT planning.
  - MRI neurogram may be used to assess for nerve root involvement but has limited utility in SBRT planning.

Radiosurgical Technique

Simulation and Treatment Planning

- Invasive stereotactic frames that attach to spinous processes (Hamilton et al. 1995; Hamilton and Lulu 1995) have fallen out of favor with the advent of noninvasive immobilization devices that allow for targeting accuracy within 1–2 mm and 1–2° (Ryu et al. 2003; Yenice et al. 2003; Li et al. 2012).
- Fluoroscopic placement of percutaneous gold fiducial markers into vertebral pedicles can be used to enhance intrafraction tumor targeting and tracking, but spinal tracking is most often sufficient.
- Insertion of a percutaneous balloon into presacral space may be considered to displace the rectum if needed for definitive treatment of complex sacral lesions.
- CT simulation with slice thickness ≤3 mm (1–1.5 mm recommended).

- MRI and/or CT myelogram should be used in patients with vertebral hardware.
- Co-registration with MRI or PET/CT images when available.
- Target volumes:
  - GTV: Gross or residual disease on CT/MRI.
  - CTV: GTV plus postoperative bed at high risk for recurrence, abnormal-appearing marrow, and adjacent normal-appearing marrow at risk for subclinical disease.
  - PTV: CTV + 1.5–2 mm margin excluding critical neural structures.

Dose Prescription

- No spine-specific randomized studies are available to provide firm recommendations for dose selection, and a clear dose-response relationship for pain control has not been established. However, there is a trend for symptomatic improvement (Ryu et al. 2003, 2007; Gerszten et al. 2006) and improved control of radioresistant histologic subtypes with increased dose (Gerszten et al. 2005a, b; Yamada et al. 2008; Zeng et al. 2021).
- No prior radiation: 16–24 Gy in 1 fraction, 20–27 Gy in 2–3 fractions, or 30–35 Gy in 5 fractions.
- Previously irradiated field: 16–20 Gy in 1 fraction, 20–27 Gy in 2 fractions, or 20–30 Gy in 5 fractions.
- Chordoma: 40 Gy in 5 fractions (UCSF experience).

Dose Delivery

- For multifraction regimens, doses are delivered daily, every other day, or twice weekly.
- Initial verification by kV X-ray or CBCT, aligned to spine or surrogate fiducial markers of position.
- Interval verification during treatment delivery with repeat kV X-ray films or CBCT for longer treatments

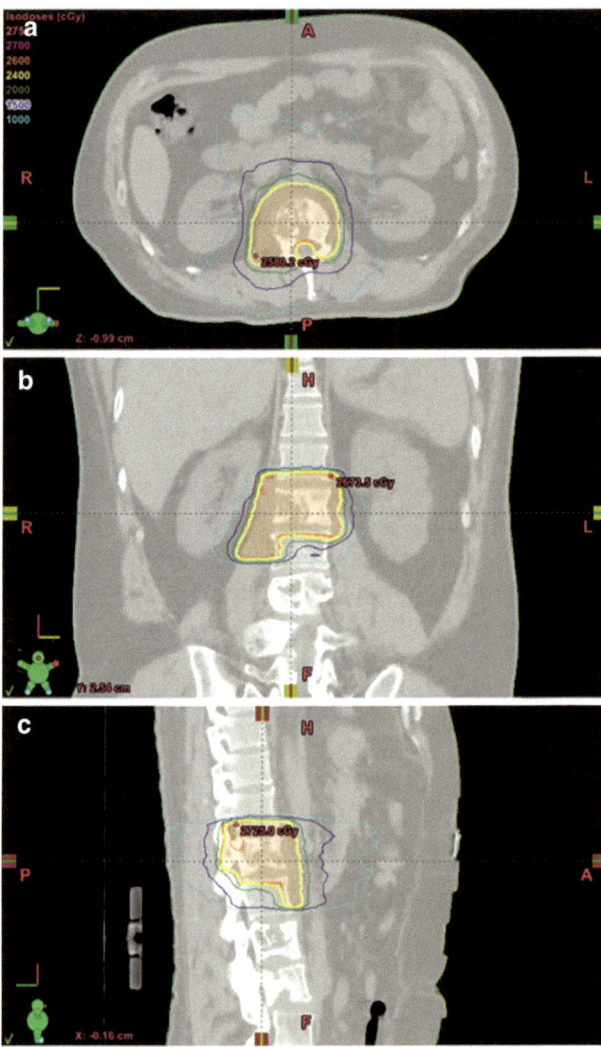

F<small>IG</small>. 4.1 SBRT for vertebral body metastasis. (a–c) Thirty-nine year-old male with stage IVC nasopharyngeal carcinoma and a painful L1 vertebral body metastasis extending to the bilateral epidural space and right psoas muscle. The metastasis was treated with rapid arc stereotactic radiosurgery to a total dose of 2400 cGy in a single fraction with 6 MV photons prescribed to the 87% isodose line

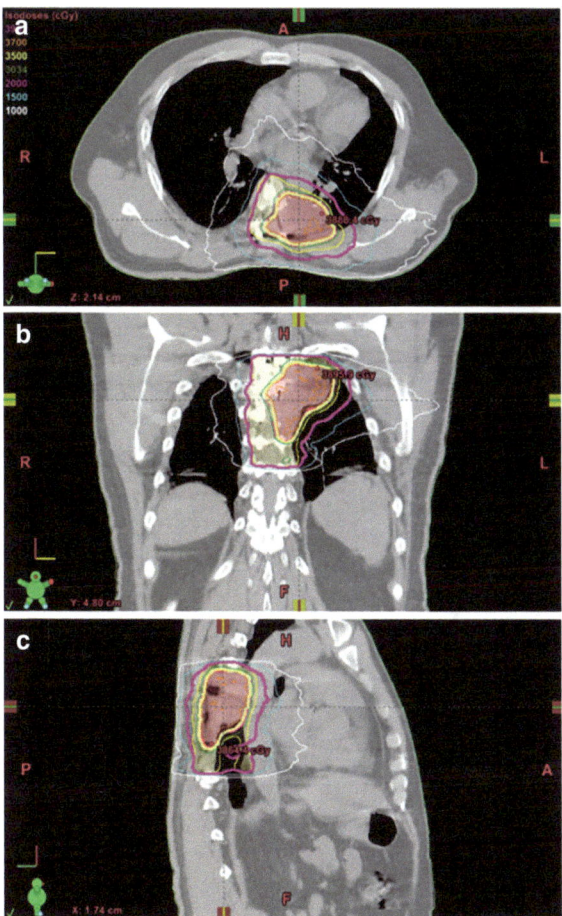

FIG. 4.2 Postoperative SBRT for primary spine tumor. (a–c) Forty-nine year-old male with a remote history of medullary thyroid cancer who subsequently developed a painful left posterior seventh rib lesion that was treated with a course of palliative radiotherapy to 3300 cGy in 11 fractions at an outside institution. The lesion continued to grow over the following 2 years, and a biopsy demonstrated chondrosarcoma. Following gross total resection and two subsequent recurrences, the GTV was treated with rapid arc stereotactic radiosurgery to a total dose of 3500 cGy in 5 fractions, with 2000 cGy to the postoperative bed, using 6 MV photons prescribed to the 88% isodose line

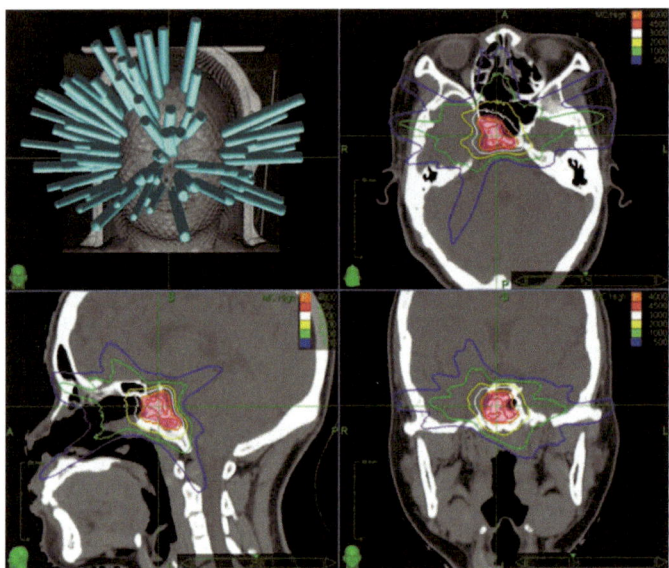

Fig. 4.3 Clival chordoma SBRT. Thirty-year-old female with a clival chordoma status post-gross total endoscopic endonasal transsphenoidal resection, followed by repeat gross total resection for a recurrence 1 year later. The tumor was treated with adjuvant robotic radiosurgery to a total dose of 4000 cGy in five daily sequential fractions with 6 MV photons prescribed to the 83% isodose line. Beam angles are shown at the top left, and proceeding clockwise are axial, coronal, and sagittal CT images with isodose lines and the PTV in red color wash

or patients unable to remain immobile (Figs. 4.1, 4.2, and 4.3).

Toxicities and Management

- Acute toxicities (≤6 weeks):
    - Low risk of acute, self-limited esophagitis, nausea/vomiting, and loose stool with treatment of cervico-

thoracic, lumbar, and sacral spinal lesions, respectively; manage with antiemetic and antidiarrheal agents.

- Cutaneous toxicities are rare, mild, and generally limited to the treatment of lesions extending into the posterior paraspinous space.
- Pain flare may occur in the days following treatment; start with reported incidence ranging from 14 to 68% and can be managed with steroids (e.g., dexamethasone) either prophylactically or as symptoms arise.
- Late toxicities (>6 weeks):
  - Vertebral body compression fracture is a fairly low-risk adverse event after conventional radiotherapy (~5%), but estimates range from 11 to 39% after spine SBRT (*vide infra*).
  - Serious late effects to the esophagus and bronchi, such as necrosis and ulceration, are rare but may require surgical intervention.
  - Late toxicities to the brachial plexus, lumbar plexus, and spinal cord, including both self-limited myelopathy and chronic progressive myelopathy, are similarly uncommon and may be mitigated with hyperbaric oxygen treatment.
  - Lhermitte's syndrome, an electric sensation running down the back into the limbs, often precedes frank neurologic deficits of radiation myelopathy.

Recommended Follow-Up

- H&P and MRI spine every 2–3 months or as clinically indicated for the first 2 years, followed by imaging every 6 months for the next 3 years, and yearly imaging thereafter.

Evidence

Dose and Technique

- Yamada et al. (2005): Noninvasive immobilization for paraspinal stereotactic or image-guided radiotherapy with setup accuracy within 2 mm. Thirty-five patients (14 primary tumors and 21 metastases) with gross disease involving the spinal canal who were either previously irradiated or treated with doses beyond conventional spinal cord tolerance. PTV = gross disease with a 1 cm margin, excluding the spinal cord. For primary treatments, median PTV dose 7000 cGy in 33 fractions with V100 of 90%; median cord Dmax 68%. In re-irradiation cases, median PTV dose 20 Gy in 5 fractions with V100 of 88%; median cord Dmax 34%. Median follow-up 11 months; no radiation myelopathy. Palliation from pain, weakness, or paresis in 90% of patients with >3 months of follow-up. LC 75 and 81% for secondary and primary malignancies, respectively.
- Chang et al. (2007): Prospective phase I/II study of SBRT for spinal metastases in 63 patients with 74 tumors treated at MDACC (30 Gy in 5 fractions or 27 Gy in 3 fractions; spinal cord Dmax ≤10 Gy). In previously radiated patients ($n = 35, 56\%$), prior dose ≤45 Gy. Median follow-up 21.3 months; no neuropathy or myelopathy. Actuarial 1-year PFS 84%. Primary mechanisms of failure limited to recurrence in adjacent bones (i.e., pedicles and posterior vertebral elements) and epidural space. Narcotic usage declined from 60 to 36% at 6 months.
- Ryu et al. (2008): Forty-nine patients with 61 separate spinal metastases treated with single-session SBRT from 10 to 16 Gy. Spinal cord limited to ≤10 Gy for ≤10% of the cord volume 6 mm superior and inferior to the treated segment. Median time to pain relief

14 days (earliest within 24 h). Complete pain relief in 46% and partial relief in 19%. Overall pain control rate for 1 year was 84%; median duration of relief 13.3 months. Trend toward increasing pain relief with ≥14 Gy. No clinically detectable late toxicity.

- Yamada et al. (2008): One-hundred three consecutive spinal metastases in 93 patients treated with 18–24 Gy in 1 fraction (median 24 Gy) prescribed to the 100% isodose line; spinal cord Dmax ≤14 Gy. Patients with high-grade cord compression, mechanical instability, and prior history of RT excluded. Median follow-up and OS both 15 months; actuarial LC 90% with median time to LF 9 months. Radiation dose, but not histologic subtype, was a significant predictor of LC. Acute toxicity limited to grade ≤2 events; no late toxicity. All patients without local failure reported durable palliation of symptoms.

- Amdur et al. (2009): Prospective phase II study of SBRT for spinal cord metastases involving 25 sites in 21 patients treated with 15 Gy in 1 fraction. Primary endpoint was toxicity; spinal cord Dmax ≤12 Gy in patients with no prior radiotherapy ($n = 9$) and ≤5 Gy for salvage cases ($n = 12$). With median follow-up of 11 months, 95% LC and 43% pain improvement, but 1-year OS 25% and PFS 5%. Acute toxicity limited to grade ≤2 dysphagia or nausea; no late toxicity.

- Cox et al. (2012): International Spine Radiosurgery Consortium consensus guidelines for target volume definitions in spine SBRT using a modified Weinstein-Boriani-Biagini system to divide vertebral body into six anatomic regions (vertebral body, bilateral pedicles, bilateral transverse processes and lamina, and spinous process). CTV should include GTV, abnormal-appearing marrow, and adjacent normal-appearing bone marrow at risk for subclinical disease. Circumferential CTV around the cord should only be used in cases of near-circumferential tumor involvement. PTV margin should be <3 mm and determined on an individual case basis depending on treatment setup and adjacent critical structures.

- Guckenberger et al. (2021): Prospective multi-institutional single-arm phase II trial of 57 patients with 63 painful nonirradiated spine metastases treated to 48.5 Gy in 10 fractions (32 patients) for long life expectancy (Mizumoto 0–4) or 35 Gy in 5 fractions (25 patients) for intermediate life expectancy (Mizumoto 5–9). Prior surgery was allowed, and patients with neurologic symptoms were excluded. Mean change in visual analog scale (VAS) pain score was −4.0 (SD 2.8) after radiation ($p < 0.001$) and remained improved throughout follow-up period (median 60 months). Net pain relief was 74% (95% CI, 65–80%). No difference in pain response rates ($p = 0.23$) or duration of pain response ($p = 0.34$) between different fractionation schemes. Median OS was 19 months, and freedom from local spinal metastasis progression was 82%. Toxicity included late grade 3 pain in 4%, progressive VCF in 14%, new VCF in 21%, and no myelopathy.

- Zelefsky et al. (2021): Prospective phase III randomized trial of 117 patients with 154 oligometastases (56.4% spine lesions) randomized 1:1 to ultrahigh single-dose radiation therapy (SDRT) to 24 Gy vs. standard hypofractionated SBRT to 27 Gy in 3 fractions. Incidence of local recurrence was improved with SDRT compared to SBRT at 2 years (2.7% vs. 9.1%) and 3 years (5.8% vs. 22%, $p = 0.0048$). Additionally, there was lower incidence of distant metastatic progression at 3 years with SDRT compared to SBRT (5.3% vs. 22.5%, $p = 0.010$). No difference in grade 2 or 3 toxicities between arms.

- Soltys et al. (2021): HyTEC systematic review of 2619 spine SBRT patients in 24 publications to provide a model of tumor control probability (TCP). To achieve 90% 2-year LC, estimated prescription doses were 20 Gy in 1 fraction, 28 Gy in 2 fractions, 33 Gy in 3 fractions, 36 Gy in 4 fractions, and 40 Gy in 5 fractions. Estimated 2-year TCPs for common dose prescriptions are 82% for 18 Gy, 90% for 20 Gy, and 96% for 24 Gy in a single fraction; 82% for 24 Gy in 2 fractions; and 78% for 27 Gy in 3 fractions. Limitations of the model include incomplete dosimetric details in published data.

SBRT Compared to Conventional EBRT

- Sprave et al. (2018): Fifty-five patients with painful spinal metastases enrolled at the University Hospital of Heidelberg in a single-institution randomized unblinded phase II trial were randomized 1:1 to SBRT 24 Gy in 1 fraction vs. 3D CRT 30 Gy in 10 fractions. Pain assessed by visual analog scale (VAS) decreased at a faster rate in the first 3 months with SBRT ($p = 0.01$), with no significant differences between arms at 3 months ($p = 0.13$), and significantly improved at 6 months with SBRT ($p = 0.002$). No significant differences in OS (mean 7.9 months), opioid usage, or acute toxicities. Incidence of new pathologic fractures at 6 months after SBRT was 27.8%.
- RTOG 0631 (presented at ASTRO 2019) (Ryu et al. 2019): Phase III randomized, multicenter trial of 339 patients with 1–3 spine metastases randomized to single-fraction spine SBRT to 16–18 Gy to involved spine segment(s) versus single-fraction conventional EBRT (cEBRT) to 8 Gy to involved spine including spine segment above and below index level (2:1 randomization). There was no difference in pain control at 3 months (40.3% SBRT vs. 57.9% cEBRT, $p = 0.99$) and no difference in adverse events.
- CCTG SC.24/TROG 17.06 (presented at ASTRO 2020) (Sahgal et al. 2020): Phase II/III randomized

multi-institutional trial of 229 patients with untreated painful spine metastases randomized 1:1 to SBRT 24 Gy in 2 fractions vs. CRT 20 Gy in 5 fractions. Patients were stratified by extra-osseous extension and radioresistant or radiosensitive type. Complete response (CR) to pain was significantly improved with SBRT at 3 months (36% vs. 14%, $p < 0.001$) and 6 months (33% vs. 16%, $p = 0.004$), which remained significantly improved on multivariable analysis. Radiation site-specific PFS at 3 months was 86% CRT vs. 92% SBRT ($p = 0.4$) and at 6 months was 69% CRT vs. 75% SBRT ($p = 0.42$). Any grade VCF rate was 17% CRT vs. 11% SBRT ($p = 0.16$).

Postoperative SBRT

- Laufer et al. (2013): MSKCC single-institution retrospective review of 186 patients who underwent "separation surgery" (epidural tumor resection for spinal cord decompression without aggressive resection of vertebral body or paraspinal tumor) followed by single-fraction (24 Gy), high-dose hypofractionated (24–30 Gy in 3 fractions), or low-dose hypofractionated (18–36 Gy in 5–6 fractions) SBRT within 2–4 weeks. There was significant improvement of local progression rate at 1 year with high-dose vs. low-dose hypofractionated SBRT (4.1% vs. 22.6%, $p = 0.04$) and no significant improvement with single-fraction SBRT (9.0%, $p = 0.09$) compared to low-dose hypofractionated SBRT.
- Redmond et al. (2017a): Consensus guidelines from 15 radiation oncologists and 5 neurosurgeons for postoperative SBRT for spinal metastases. Indications include radioresistant primary, 1–2 levels of adjacent disease, and prior overlapping radiation therapy. Contraindications include involvement of more than

three contiguous vertebral bodies, complete spinal cord injury, and postoperative Bilsky grade 3 residual.

- Redmond et al. (2017b): Consensus contouring guidelines for postoperative spine SBRT recommend CTV inclusion of the entire GTV, preoperative extent of bony and epidural disease, and immediately adjacent bony anatomic compartments; hardware should not be included unless involved; consider 5 mm expansion beyond paraspinal disease and craniocaudally for epidural disease; and use of circumferential CTV only in preoperative near or total circumferential epidural involvement.

- Alghamdi et al. (2019): Sunnybrook single-institution retrospective review of 47 patients with 83 spinal segments treated with postoperative SBRT. Median dose was 24 Gy in 2 fractions. Median follow-up was 11.7 months per patient. One-year local failure and OS rates were 17% and 55%, respectively. Predictors for LC on MVA were grade of postoperative epidural disease and longer time from prior radiotherapy (for those undergoing re-irradiation). Toxicity included one patient with radiculopathy after two prior courses of radiation, three VCF, and no myelopathy.

- Redmond et al. (2020): Johns Hopkins single-institution phase II prospective study of 35 targets in 33 patients treated with SBRT 30 Gy in 5 fractions within 16 weeks of surgical resection of spinal metastasis. Local control at 1 year was 90.0% (95% CI, 76–98%). Local failures all occurred epidurally and at a median of 3.5 months. There were no grade 3 or higher toxicities and no incidences of wound dehiscence or hardware failure. There was also improvement in epidural disease after SBRT measured by Bilsky grade.

- Blakaj et al. (2021): Ohio State University single-institution retrospective review of 63 patients who underwent spine surgery followed by SBRT with median follow-up of 12.5 months. Median SBRT dose was 27 Gy in 3 fractions. One-year LC was 81%, which was improved for patients treated within 40 days of surgery (94% vs. 75%, $p = 0.03$) and underwent preoperative embolization (88% vs. 76%, $p = 0.037$). Predictors for LC on MVA were time from surgery to SBRT, preoperative embolization, and higher biologically equivalent dose. One-year PFS and OS were 56% and 60%, respectively. Acute grade 1–2 toxicity rate was 28%, and there were no high-grade late toxicities.

Spinal Cord Compression and Retreatment

- Milker-Zabel et al. (2003): Eighteen patients with 19 previously irradiated spinal cord metastases (median dose 38 Gy) re-treated due to progressive pain ($n = 16$) or neurologic symptoms ($n = 12$). Median time to re-treatment 17.7 months. Five patients treated with fractionated conformal radiotherapy (FCRT), and 14 treated with IMRT; all immobilized for extracranial stereotaxy. Median re-treatment dose 39.6 Gy in 2 Gy fractions. After a median of 12 months of follow-up, OS 65%, LC 95%, pain relief 81%, and neurologic improvement 42%. Tumor size unchanged in 84% of cases. No clinical late toxicity.
- Gerszten et al. (2007): Single-institution cohort of 393 patients with spinal cord compression treated with 12.5–25 Gy robot-assisted SBRT in 1 fraction (mean 20 Gy) and followed prospectively. Five hundred metastases, 67% previously treated with EBRT. Long-term improvement in pain for 86% of patients; 84% (30 of 35) with progressive neurological deficit experienced clinical improvement. LC was 90 and 88% for primary and salvage SBRT, respectively. No reports of radiation myelopathy.
- Sahgal et al. (2009): Single-institution retrospective review of 39 consecutive patients with 60 paraspinal

metastases treated with robot-assisted SBRT. Median dose 24 Gy in 3 fractions prescribed to the 60–67% isodose line. Sixty-two percent of lesions previously treated with EBRT. Median OS 21 months; 1- and 2-year PFP rates were 85% and 69%, respectively. For re-irradiation cases, 1-year PFP was 96%. No significant differences in OS or PFP between salvage and de novo treatments. No reports of radiation-induced myelopathy or radiculopathy in the 39 cases with ≥6 months' follow-up. All patients with local failure experienced worsening of pain; all others stable at best, but no standardized pain quantification used.

- Hashmi et al. (2016): Multi-institutional retrospective study of 215 patients with 247 spinal targets treated at seven institutions with re-irradiation SBRT after previous conventional EBRT. Median re-irradiation dose was 18 Gy in 1 fraction. Sixty percent of spinal targets were treated with a single fraction to median 16.6 Gy and 40% were treated with multiple fractions to median 24 Gy in 3 fractions. Median time from conventional EBRT to re-irradiation SBRT was 13.5 months, and median follow-up was 8.1 months. Six- and 12-month OS rates were 64% and 48%, respectively, while 6- and 12-month LC rates were 93% and 83%, respectively. MVA revealed KPS <70 prognostic for worse survival and single-fraction SBRT predictive for LC. VCF rate was 4.5%, and there were no cases of radiation myelopathy.

- Myrehaug et al. (2017): International Stereotactic Radiosurgery Society guidelines for spine re-treatment with SBRT as a treatment option following conventional EBRT or previous SBRT (level III evidence), and if concerns for epidural spinal cord compression or mechanical stability, a spine surgeon should be consulted before the patient undergoes SBRT (level II evidence). Included systematic review of 9 studies of

411 spine segments re-irradiated with SBRT. Median local control at 1 year was 76% (range 66–90%) for SBRT following prior conventional EBRT. Epidural disease was the most common site of progression (38–63%). Pain control was achieved in 65–81% of cases. Toxicity included VCF rate of 12% and radiation myelopathy rate of 1.2% with no other grade 3–4 toxicities.

Chordoma and Other Primary Tumors of the Spine and Skull Base

- Martin et al. (2007): Twenty-eight patients with chordoma ($n = 18$) or chondrosarcoma ($n = 10$) of the skull base treated with Gamma Knife SRS as either primary ($n = 2$) or adjuvant treatment. Twenty-two patients previously received fractionated radiotherapy prior to radiosurgery (mean dose 65 Gy and 75 CGE). Mean tumor volume at SRS 9.8 cm³. Median dose to the tumor margin 16 Gy in 1 fraction (range 10.5–25 Gy) prescribed to the 50% isodose line in all but 1 patient. Transient acute toxicity in 1 patient. Median follow-up 7.7 years. Five-year actuarial LC for chondrosarcoma $80 \pm 10\%$; chordoma actuarial LC and survival $63 \pm 10\%$ at both 5 and 10 years. No significant factors identified for tumor control.
- Henderson et al. (2009): Eighteen chordoma patients treated with stereotactic robotic radiosurgery; 44% mobile spine, 39% clivus, and 17% sacral tumors. Median tumor volume 128 cm³ treated with a median dose of 35 Gy in 5 fractions; salvage cases treated with 28 Gy in 4 fractions. Five-year LC 59%, OS 74%, and DSS 89%. No improvement in pain or quality of life. Recommendation for 40 Gy in 5 fractions to gross tumor and at least a 1 cm margin based on modeling with α/β of 2.45 for chordoma.

- North American Gamma Knife Consortium (Kano et al. 2011): Seventy-one patients status post-SRS for chordoma from six institutions. Median target volume 7.1 cm³, and median marginal dose 15 Gy. Five-year actuarial OS 80%; 93% for patients with no prior fractionated RT (n = 50), and 43% for prior RT group (n = 21). Younger age, longer interval between initial diagnosis and SRS, no prior RT, <2 cranial nerve deficits, and smaller tumor volume were significantly associated with longer survival. Five-year overall LC 66%; 69% for no prior RT, and 62% for prior RT. Older age, prior RT, and large tumor volume all significantly associated with worse tumor control. Thirty percent of patients with pretreatment neurologic deficits experienced improvement; median time to response 4.6 months.
- Jiang et al. (2012): Twenty patients with chordoma treated with stereotactic robotic radiosurgery (11 primary adjuvant therapy, 9 salvage); 65% clival lesions. Average tumor volume 16 cm³; mean marginal dose of 32.5 Gy in 1–5 fractions to the 79% isodose line. With a median follow-up of 34 months, LC 55%; 82% in primary adjuvant cases, and 29% in salvage cases. Five-year OS 52.5%. Status of symptoms not reported.
- Yamada et al. (2013): Twenty-four patients with chordoma of the sacrum (n = 10) and mobile spine (n = 14) treated with single-fraction SRS (median dose 24 Gy, with median V100 95%). Treatment given in both the adjuvant (n = 7) and neoadjuvant setting (n = 13), although only six patients proceeded to surgery. Seven patients treated for postoperative recurrence. With a median follow-up of 24 months, LC 95%; 1 case of progression 11 months after SRS. Toxicity limited to 1 case of sciatic neuropathy and 1 case of vocal cord paralysis. Status of symptoms not reported.
- Vasudevan et al. (2017): UCSF single-institution retrospective review of 20 patients with chordoma or chon-

drosarcoma treated with fractionated SBRT in 5 fractions to median dose of 37.5 Gy (range 24–40 Gy) with median follow-up of 28 months. Overall LRFS was 90% and 3-year LRFS was 88.67% (95% CI 61–97%). One-year OS was 93.8% (95% CI 63–99%). Acute toxicity occurred in nine patients (45%) and late toxicity in two patients, including one grade 5 radiation vasculopathy in a previously irradiated patient.

- Jin et al. (2019): MSKCC single-institution retrospective review of 35 patients treated for de novo chordoma of the spine and sacrum with single-fraction SBRT to median 24 Gy (range 18–24 Gy). Twelve patients (34%) received definitive SBRT, and 23 patients (66%) received surgery and SBRT. Local recurrence-free survival (LRFS) rates at 3 and 5 years were 86.2% and 80.5%, respectively. For the 32 patients receiving 24 Gy, LRFS rates at 3 and 5 years were 96.3% and 89.9%, respectively. OS rates at 3 and 5 years were 90.0% and 84.3%, respectively. Acute grade 2 toxicity rate was 40%, and long-term grade 2 and grade 3 toxicity was 31% and 20%, respectively.

Vertebral Body Compression Fracture (VCF)

- Rose et al. (2009): 62 patients with 71 spinal metastases treated with single-fraction SBRT (median 24 Gy); predominance of lytic spinal lesions (65%). With a median follow-up of 13 months, VCF occurred in 27 (39%) treated sites after a median time of 25 months. HR for VCF: osteolytic tumors 3.8; >40% vertebral body involvement 3.9; and lesions located from T10 through the sacrum 4.6.
- Sahgal et al. (2013a): Pooled retrospective study of 252 patients with 410 spinal segments treated with SBRT at MDACC, Cleveland Clinic, and University of Toronto. Median follow-up and OS of 11.5 and

16 months, respectively. Twenty-seven new VCFs and 30 cases of VCF progression (overall incidence 14%). Median time to VCF 2.46 months, with 65% of events occurring in the first 4 months. Dose per fraction identified as a significant predictor of VCF on univariate and multivariate analysis; baseline VCF, lytic tumors, and spinal deformity all significant on multivariate analysis. Relative to ≤19 Gy per fraction, the HR for VCF with ≥24 Gy and 20–23 Gy per fraction was 5.25 and 4.91, respectively.

- Jawad et al. (2016): Multi-institution retrospective study from Elekta Spine SBRT Research Consortium of 594 malignant spine tumors treated with SBRT in 1–5 fractions with a median follow-up of 10.1 months. Overall LC was 80%. Thirty-four patients (5.7%) developed new (3%) or progressive (2.7%) VCF after SBRT at a median time of 3 months. Preexisting VCF, solitary metastasis, and prescription dose of >38.4 Gy were predictive of VCF on MVA. Solitary metastasis and lack of MRI use for target delineation were predictive of new VCF on MVA.

- Virk et al. (2017): MSKCC single-institution retrospective study of 323 patients who underwent 24 Gy in a single-fraction SBRT to spine. Patients with local recurrence after SBRT were excluded from analysis. Median survival was 11 months. Twenty-six (7.2%) patients developed VCF at 5 years, of which 62% was de novo and 38% was progression of existing fractures. Median time to VCF was 13.2 months. Treatment of VCF consisted of kyphoplasty alone (six patients), surgery alone (ten patients), or both kyphoplasty and surgery (ten patients). For patients who did not have previous stabilization before SBRT, there was a correlation between higher SINS score and time to VCF ($p < 0.001$).

Pain Flare

- Chiang et al. (2013): Sunnybrook single-institution prospective study of 41 steroid-naïve patients receiving spine SBRT to define the incidence of pain flare. Twenty-eight patients (68.3%) experienced pain flare as defined as a two-point increase of worst pain score without decreasing analgesics (53.5%), increasing analgesic intake by 25% without change in pain score (17.9%), or initiation of steroids (28.6%). Pain flare occurred most commonly on day 1 after completing SBRT. Higher KPS and cervical or lumbar spine segments had significantly higher probability for pain flare on MVA.
- Pan et al. (2014): Secondary analysis of 195 patients enrolled at MDACC in single-institution prospective phase I/II trials of single-fraction (18 Gy or 24 Gy) and multiple-fraction (30 Gy in 5 fractions or 27 Gy in 3 fractions) spine SBRT. Forty-four patients (23%) experienced pain flare assessed by increase in pain score or medication changes. Median time to pain flare was 5 days after treatment start. Single-fraction treatment was predictive, and increasing number of fractions was protective of pain flare on MVA ($p = 0.005$).
- Khan et al. (2015): Sunnybrook single-institution sequential prospective study of 47 patients treated with spine SBRT evaluating dexamethasone 4 or 8 mg 1 h prior to SBRT followed by daily dose for 4 days after completing SBRT. Nine patients (19.2%) experienced a pain flare as defined by a previous study from the same institution (Chiang et al. 2013), of whom 6 (25%) took dexamethasone 4 mg and 3 (13%) took 8 mg ($p = 0.46$). However, dexamethasone 8 mg use was associated with higher Brief Pain Inventory (BPI) scores for walking ability ($p = 0.005$) and relations with others ($p = 0.035$) compared to 4 mg.
- Balagamwala et al. (2018): Cleveland Clinic single-institution retrospective study of 507 lesions in 348

patients treated with single-fraction spine SBRT (median dose 15 Gy). Seventy-three treatments (14.4%) resulted in a pain flare defined by increase in pain within 7 days requiring initiation of steroids. Higher KPS ($p = 0.04$), female gender ($p = 0.01$), higher prescription dose ($p = 0.02$), and cervical/thoracic location ($p = 0.05$) were associated with increased risk of pain flare on MVA.

Late Toxicity

- Ryu et al. (2007): Retrospective analysis of 230 lesions treated with single-fraction SBRT to the gross tumor plus vertebral body and pedicles and/or posterior elements in 177 patients without a history of prior radiotherapy to the spine. Prescription ranged from 8 to 18 Gy to the 90% isodose line; no PTV margin; spinal cord volume defined as 6 mm superior and inferior to the target. Among the patients treated with 18 Gy, the average dose to the 10% spinal cord volume was 9.8 ± 1.5 Gy. Median follow-up 6.4 months; 1-year survival 49%. One case of radiation myelopathy among the 86 patients alive >1 year after treatment.
- Gomez et al. (2009): Retrospective analysis of 119 paraspinal thoracic sites treated with single-fraction SBRT (median dose 24 Gy) in 114 patients. Median Dmax to esophagi and bronchi was 12.5 Gy and 11 Gy, respectively. At a median follow-up of 11.6 months, seven episodes of grade ≥ 2 esophageal toxicity (one of which required gastric pull-up for fistula formation), and two cases of grade ≥ 2 bronchial toxicity; no cases of pneumonitis.
- Sahgal et al. (2010): Dosimetric report of radiation-induced myelopathy in five patients after primary SBRT for spinal tumors. Radiation myelopathy observed with Dmax of 10.6–14.8 Gy in 1 fraction,

25.6 Gy in 2 fractions, and 30.9 Gy in 3 fractions to the thecal sac. When compared to dosimetric data from 19 patients without spinal cord myelopathy after SBRT, there was a significant interaction between patient subsets based on normalized BED. Modeling with α/β value of 2 for spinal cord late effect and 10 for tumor effect suggests that 10 Gy in 1 fraction and up to 35 Gy_2 in 5 fractions carry a low risk of radiation-induced myelopathy.

- Sahgal et al. (2012): Dosimetric report of radiation-induced myelopathy after salvage SBRT in five patients who initially received conventional EBRT to the spine (median 40 Gy in 20 fractions). When compared to a group of 14 salvage patients without radiation myelopathy, the mean EQD2 maximum point dose (P_{max}) to the thecal sac was significantly higher in those with radiation myelopathy (67.4 Gy vs. 20 Gy), as was the total P_{max} (105.8 Gy vs. 62.3 Gy). Modeling suggests that SBRT given at least 5 months after conventional palliative radiotherapy with a re-irradiation thecal sac P_{max} EQD2 of 20–25 Gy appears to be safe provided that the total P_{max} EQD2 does not exceed 70 Gy, and the thecal sac P_{max} EQD2 comprises no more than one-half of the total EQD2.

- Sahgal et al. (2013b): Dosimetric analysis of 9 cases of radiation myelopathy (RM) occurring after spine SBRT compared to 66 patients with no RM after spine SBRT from multiple institutions. Biologically equivalent doses were calculated at 2 Gy equivalent with $\alpha/\beta = 2$ Gy, and a logistic regression model was used to estimate the probability of RM. A $\leq 5\%$ risk of RM was observed when limiting the thecal sac point maximum dose to 12.4 Gy in 1 fraction, 17.0 Gy in 2 fractions, 20.3 Gy in 3 fractions, 23.0 Gy in 4 fractions, and 25.3 Gy in 5 fractions.

- Sahgal et al. (2019): HyTEC review and modeling of published retrospective studies on radiation myelopathy after de novo and re-irradiation spine SBRT. For de novo spine SBRT, D_{max} to thecal sac of 12.4–14.0 Gy in 1 fraction, 17.0 Gy in 2 fractions, 20.3 Gy in 3 fractions, 23.0 Gy in 4 fractions, and 25.3 Gy in 5 fractions are likely associated with a 1–5% risk of radiation myelopathy. For re-irradiation spine SBRT, cumulative thecal sac EQD2$_2$ D_{max} < 70 Gy, re-irradiation EQD2$_2$ D_{max} < 25 Gy, re-irradiation to cumulative D_{max} ratio <0.5, and minimum time interval of 5 months are likely associated with low risk of radiation myelopathy. Due to low number of reported radiation myelopathy cases, future studies with larger cohorts are needed to refine estimates of radiation myelopathy risk and should report specific dosimetric parameters (i.e., D_{max}, $D_{0.03cc}$, $D_{0.1cc}$, D_{1cc}, $D_{50\%}$).

References

Alghamdi M, Sahgal A, Soliman H, Myrehaug S, Yang VXD, Das S, et al. Postoperative stereotactic body radiotherapy for spinal metastases and the impact of epidural disease grade. Neurosurgery. 2019;85:E1111–8.

Amdur RJ, Bennett J, Olivier K, Wallace A, Morris CG, Liu C, et al. A prospective, phase II study demonstrating the potential value and limitation of radiosurgery for spine metastases. Am J Clin Oncol. 2009;32:515–20.

Balagamwala EH, Naik M, Reddy CA, Angelov L, Suh JH, Djemil T, et al. Pain flare after stereotactic radiosurgery for spine metastases. J Radiosurg SBRT. 2018;5:99–105.

Barzilai O, DiStefano N, Lis E, Yamada Y, Lovelock DM, Fontanella AN, et al. Safety and utility of kyphoplasty prior to spine stereotactic radiosurgery for metastatic tumors: a clinical and dosimetric analysis. J Neurosurg Spine. 2018;28:72–8.

Blakaj DM, Palmer JD, Dibs K, Olausson A, Bourekas EC, Boulter D, et al. Postoperative stereotactic body radiotherapy for spinal metastasis and predictors of local control. Neurosurgery. 2021;88:1021–7.

Chang EL, Shiu AS, Mendel E, Mathews LA, Mahajan A, Allen PK, et al. Phase I/II study of stereotactic body radiotherapy for spinal metastasis and its pattern of failure. J Neurosurg Spine. 2007;7:151–60.

Chiang A, Zeng L, Zhang L, Lochray F, Korol R, Loblaw A, et al. Pain flare is a common adverse event in steroid-naïve patients after spine stereotactic body radiation therapy: a prospective clinical trial. Int J Radiat Oncol Biol Phys. 2013;86:638–42.

Cox BW, Spratt DE, Lovelock M, Bilsky MH, Lis E, Ryu S, et al. International Spine Radiosurgery Consortium consensus guidelines for target volume definition in spinal stereotactic radiosurgery. Int J Radiat Oncol Biol Phys. 2012;83:e597–605.

Cruz JP, Sahgal A, Whyne C, Fehlings MG, Smith R. Tumor extravasation following a cement augmentation procedure for vertebral compression fracture in metastatic spinal disease. J Neurosurg Spine. 2014;21:372–7.

Gerszten PC, Burton SA, Ozhasoglu C, Vogel WJ, Welch WC, Baar J, et al. Stereotactic radiosurgery for spinal metastases from renal cell carcinoma. J Neurosurg Spine. 2005a;3:288–95.

Gerszten PC, Burton SA, Quinn AE, Agarwala SS, Kirkwood JM. Radiosurgery for the treatment of spinal melanoma metastases. Stereotact Funct Neurosurg. 2005b;83:213–21.

Gerszten PC, Burton SA, Belani CP, Ramalingam S, Friedland DM, Ozhasoglu C, et al. Radiosurgery for the treatment of spinal lung metastases. Cancer. 2006;107:2653–61.

Gerszten PC, Burton SA, Ozhasoglu C, Welch WC. Radiosurgery for spinal metastases: clinical experience in 500 cases from a single institution. Spine. 2007;32:193–9.

Gomez DR, Hunt MA, Jackson A, O'Meara WP, Bukanova EN, Zelefsky MJ, et al. Low rate of thoracic toxicity in palliative paraspinal single-fraction stereotactic body radiation therapy. Radiother Oncol. 2009;93:414–8.

Guckenberger M, Mantel F, Sweeney RA, Hawkins M, Belderbos J, Ahmed M, et al. Long-term results of dose-intensified fractionated stereotactic body radiation therapy (SBRT) for painful spinal metastases. Int J Radiat Oncol Biol Phys. 2021;110(2):348–57.

Hamilton AJ, Lulu BA. A prototype device for linear accelerator-based extracranial radiosurgery. Acta Neurochir Suppl. 1995;63:40–3.

Hamilton AJ, Lulu BA, Fosmire H, Stea B, Cassady JR. Preliminary clinical experience with linear accelerator-based spinal stereotactic radiosurgery. Neurosurgery. 1995;36:311–9.

Hashmi A, Guckenberger M, Kersh R, Gerszten PC, Mantel F, Grills IS, et al. Re-irradiation stereotactic body radiotherapy for spinal metastases: a multi-institutional outcome analysis. J Neurosurg Spine. 2016;25:646–53.

Henderson FC, McCool K, Seigle J, Jean W, Harter W, Gagnon GJ. Treatment of chordomas with CyberKnife: Georgetown University experience and treatment recommendations. Neurosurgery. 2009;64:A44–53.

Husain ZA, Sahgal A, De Salles A, Funaro M, Glover J, Hayashi M, et al. Stereotactic body radiotherapy for de novo spinal metastases: systematic review. J Neurosurg Spine. 2017;27:295–302.

Jawad MS, Fahim DK, Gerszten PC, Flickinger JC, Sahgal A, Grills IS, et al. Vertebral compression fractures after stereotactic body radiation therapy: a large, multi-institutional, multinational evaluation. J Neurosurg Spine. 2016;24:928–36.

Jiang B, Veeravagu A, Lee M, Harsh GR, Lieberson RE, Bhatti I, et al. Management of intracranial and extracranial chordomas with CyberKnife stereotactic radiosurgery. J Clin Neurosci. 2012;19:1101–6.

Jin CJ, Berry-Candelario J, Reiner AS, Laufer I, Higginson DS, Schmitt AM, et al. Long-term outcomes of high-dose single-fraction radiosurgery for chordomas of the spine and sacrum. J Neurosurg Spine. 2019:1–10.

Kano H, Iqbal FO, Sheehan J, Mathieu D, Seymour ZA, Niranjan A, et al. Stereotactic radiosurgery for chordoma: a report from the North American Gamma Knife Consortium. Neurosurgery. 2011;68:379–89.

Khan L, Chiang A, Zhang L, Thibault I, Bedard G, Wong E, et al. Prophylactic dexamethasone effectively reduces the incidence of pain flare following spine stereotactic body radiotherapy (SBRT): a prospective observational study. Support Care Cancer. 2015;23:2937–43.

Laufer I, Iorgulescu JB, Chapman T, Lis E, Shi W, Zhang Z, et al. Local disease control for spinal metastases following "separation surgery" and adjuvant hypofractionated or high-dose single-fraction stereotactic radiosurgery: outcome analysis in 186 patients. J Neurosurg Spine. 2013;18:207–14.

Li W, Sahgal A, Foote M, Millar B-A, Jaffray DA, Letourneau D. Impact of immobilization on intrafraction motion for spine stereotactic body radiotherapy using cone beam computed tomography. Int J Radiat Oncol Biol Phys. 2012;84:520–6.

Linstadt DE, Nakamura JL. Spinal cord tumors. Leibel and Phillips textbook of radiation oncology. Elsevier; 2010. p. 509–22.

Lis E, Laufer I, Barzilai O, Yamada Y, Karimi S, McLaughlin L, et al. Change in the cross-sectional area of the thecal sac following balloon kyphoplasty for pathological vertebral compression fractures prior to spine stereotactic radiosurgery. J Neurosurg Spine. 2018;30:111–8.

Lo SS, Sahgal A, Wang JZ, Mayr NA, Sloan A, Mendel E, et al. Stereotactic body radiation therapy for spinal metastases. Discov Med. 2010;9:289–96.

Lutz S, Balboni T, Jones J, Lo S, Petit J, Rich SE, et al. Palliative radiation therapy for bone metastases: update of an ASTRO evidence-based guideline. Pract Radiat Oncol. 2017;7:4–12.

Martin JJ, Niranjan A, Kondziolka D, Flickinger JC, Lozanne KA, Lunsford LD. Radiosurgery for chordomas and chondrosarcomas of the skull base. J Neurosurg. 2007;107:758–64.

Milker-Zabel S, Zabel A, Thilmann C, Schlegel W, Wannenmacher M, Debus J. Clinical results of retreatment of vertebral bone metastases by stereotactic conformal radiotherapy and intensity-modulated radiotherapy. Int J Radiat Oncol Biol Phys. 2003;55:162–7.

Mizumoto M, Harada H, Asakura H, Hashimoto T, Furutani K, Hashii H, et al. Radiotherapy for patients with metastases to the spinal column: a review of 603 patients at Shizuoka Cancer Center Hospital. Int J Radiat Oncol Biol Phys. 2011;79:208–13.

Myrehaug S, Sahgal A, Hayashi M, Levivier M, Ma L, Martinez R, et al. Reirradiation spine stereotactic body radiation therapy for spinal metastases: systematic review. J Neurosurg Spine. 2017;27:428–35.

Pan HY, Allen PK, Wang XS, Chang EL, Rhines LD, Tatsui CE, et al. Incidence and predictive factors of pain flare after spine stereotactic body radiation therapy: secondary analysis of phase 1/2 trials. Int J Radiat Oncol Biol Phys. 2014;90:870–6.

Redmond KJ, Lo SS, Soltys SG, Yamada Y, Barani IJ, Brown PD, et al. Consensus guidelines for postoperative stereotactic body radiation therapy for spinal metastases: results of an international survey. J Neurosurg Spine. 2017a;26:299–306.

Redmond KJ, Robertson S, Lo SS, Soltys SG, Ryu S, McNutt T, et al. Consensus contouring guidelines for postoperative stereotactic body radiation therapy for metastatic solid tumor malignancies to the spine. Int J Radiat Oncol Biol Phys. 2017b;97:64–74.

Redmond KJ, Sciubba D, Khan M, Gui C, Lo S-FL, Gokaslan ZL, et al. A phase 2 study of post-operative stereotactic body radiation therapy (SBRT) for solid tumor spine metastases. Int J Radiat Oncol Biol Phys. 2020;106:261–8.

Rose PS, Laufer I, Boland PJ, Hanover A, Bilsky MH, Yamada J, et al. Risk of fracture after single fraction image-guided intensity-modulated radiation therapy to spinal metastases. J Clin Oncol. 2009;27:5075–9.

Ryu S, Fang Yin F, Rock J, Zhu J, Chu A, Kagan E, et al. Image-guided and intensity-modulated radiosurgery for patients with spinal metastasis. Cancer. 2003;97:2013–8.

Ryu S, Jin J-Y, Jin R, Rock J, Ajlouni M, Movsas B, et al. Partial volume tolerance of the spinal cord and complications of single-dose radiosurgery. Cancer. 2007;109:628–36.

Ryu S, Jin R, Jin J-Y, Chen Q, Rock J, Anderson J, et al. Pain control by image-guided radiosurgery for solitary spinal metastasis. J Pain Symptom Manag. 2008;35:292–8.

Ryu S, Deshmukh S, Timmerman RD, Movsas B, Gerszten PC, Yin FF, et al. Radiosurgery compared to external beam radiotherapy for localized spine metastasis: phase III results of NRG oncology/rtog 0631. Int J Radiat Oncol Biol Phys. 2019;105:S2–3.

Sahgal A, Ames C, Chou D, Ma L, Huang K, Xu W, et al. Stereotactic body radiotherapy is effective salvage therapy for patients with prior radiation of spinal metastases. Int J Radiat Oncol Biol Phys. 2009;74:723–31.

Sahgal A, Ma L, Gibbs I, Gerszten PC, Ryu S, Soltys S, et al. Spinal cord tolerance for stereotactic body radiotherapy. Int J Radiat Oncol Biol Phys. 2010;77:548–53.

Sahgal A, Ma L, Weinberg V, Gibbs IC, Chao S, Chang U-K, et al. Reirradiation human spinal cord tolerance for stereotactic body radiotherapy. Int J Radiat Oncol Biol Phys. 2012;82:107–16.

Sahgal A, Atenafu EG, Chao S, Al-Omair A, Boehling N, Balagamwala EH, et al. Vertebral compression fracture after spine stereotactic body radiotherapy: a multi-institutional analysis with a focus on radiation dose and the spinal instability neoplastic score. J Clin Oncol. 2013a;31:3426–31.

Sahgal A, Weinberg V, Ma L, Chang E, Chao S, Muacevic A, et al. Probabilities of radiation myelopathy specific to stereotactic

118   J. Chew et al.

body radiation therapy to guide safe practice. Int J Radiat Oncol Biol Phys. 2013b;85:341–7.

Sahgal A, Chang JH, Ma L, Marks LB, Milano MT, Medin P, et al. Spinal cord dose tolerance to stereotactic body radiation therapy. Int J Radiat Oncol Biol Phys. 2019;110(1):124–36.

Sahgal A, Myrehaug SD, Siva S, Masucci L, Foote MC, Brundage M, et al. CCTG SC.24/TROG 17.06: a randomized phase II/III study comparing 24Gy in 2 stereotactic body radiotherapy (SBRT) fractions versus 20Gy in 5 conventional palliative radiotherapy (CRT) fractions for patients with painful spinal metastases. Int J Radiat Oncol Biol Phys. 2020;108:1397–8.

Sciubba DM, Pennington Z, Colman MW, Goodwin CR, Laufer I, Patt JC, et al. Spinal metastases 2021: a review of the current state of the art and future directions. Spine J. 2021;21(9):1414–29.

Soltys SG, Grimm J, Milano MT, Xue J, Sahgal A, Yorke E, et al. Stereotactic body radiation therapy for spinal metastases: tumor control probability analyses and recommended reporting standards. Int J Radiat Oncol Biol Phys. 2021;110(1):112–23.

Sprave T, Verma V, Förster R, Schlampp I, Bruckner T, Bostel T, et al. Randomized phase II trial evaluating pain response in patients with spinal metastases following stereotactic body radiotherapy versus three-dimensional conformal radiotherapy. Radiother Oncol. 2018;128:274–82.

Vasudevan HN, Raleigh DR, Johnson J, Garsa AA, Theodosopoulos PV, Aghi MK, et al. Management of chordoma and chondrosarcoma with fractionated stereotactic radiotherapy. Front Surg. 2017;4:35.

Virk MS, Han JE, Reiner AS, McLaughlin LA, Sciubba DM, Lis E, et al. Frequency of symptomatic vertebral body compression fractures requiring intervention following single-fraction stereotactic radiosurgery for spinal metastases. Neurosurg Focus. 2017;42:E8.

Yamada Y, Lovelock DM, Yenice KM, Bilsky MH, Hunt MA, Zatcky J, et al. Multifractionated image-guided and stereotactic intensity-modulated radiotherapy of paraspinal tumors: a preliminary report. Int J Radiat Oncol Biol Phys. 2005;62:53–61.

Yamada Y, Bilsky MH, Lovelock DM, Venkatraman ES, Toner S, Johnson J, et al. High-dose, single-fraction image-guided intensity-modulated radiotherapy for metastatic spinal lesions. Int J Radiat Oncol Biol Phys. 2008;71:484–90.

Yamada Y, Laufer I, Cox BW, Lovelock DM, Maki RG, Zatcky JM, et al. Preliminary results of high-dose single-fraction radiotherapy for the management of chordomas of the spine and sacrum. Neurosurgery. 2013;73:673–80. discussion 680

Yenice KM, Lovelock DM, Hunt MA, Lutz WR, Fournier-Bidoz N, Hua C-H, et al. CT image-guided intensity-modulated therapy for paraspinal tumors using stereotactic immobilization. Int J Radiat Oncol Biol Phys. 2003;55:583–93.

Zelefsky MJ, Yamada Y, Greco C, Lis E, Schöder H, Lobaugh S, et al. Phase 3 multi-center, prospective, randomized trial comparing single-dose 24 Gy radiation therapy to a 3-fraction SBRT regimen in the treatment of oligometastatic cancer. Int J Radiat Oncol Biol Phys. 2021;110(3):672–9.

Zeng KL, Sahgal A, Husain ZA, Myrehaug S, Tseng C-L, Detsky J, et al. Local control and patterns of failure for "Radioresistant" spinal metastases following stereotactic body radiotherapy compared to a "Radiosensitive" reference. J Neuro-Oncol. 2021;152:173–82.

Chapter 5
Head and Neck

Christina Phuong and Jason W. Chan

Pearls

- Treatment options are limited for patients who experience locoregional recurrences and/or second primary tumors in previously irradiated regions of the head and neck.
- Isolated locoregional recurrences occur in 30–40% of patients irradiated for advanced head and neck cancers.
- Second primary head and neck cancers occur in roughly 15% of patients with head and neck squamous cell carcinoma (HNSCC).
- SBRT is an accepted treatment option for re-irradiation of small targets in the head and neck and for oligometastases of head and neck primary origin.

C. Phuong · J. W. Chan (✉)
Department of Radiation Oncology, University of California, San Francisco, San Francisco, CA, USA
e-mail: Christina.Phuong@ucsf.edu; Jason.w.chan@ucsf.edu

121

R. A. Sethi et al. (eds.), *Handbook of Evidence-Based Stereotactic Radiosurgery and Stereotactic Body Radiotherapy*,
https://doi.org/10.1007/978-3-031-33156-5_5

- At present, SBRT has no widely accepted role in the definitive treatment of newly diagnosed, nonmetastatic head and neck cancer.
- The potentially serious risks of SBRT should be cautiously weighed against the competing risks of symptomatic tumor progression and the feasibility and efficacy of alternative treatment options.

Workup

- H&P, including performance status, HPV status, smoking and alcohol history, prior history of treatment to the head and neck
- Review of symptoms, including:
  - Bleeding
  - Pain
  - Weight loss/nutritional status
  - Preexisting dysphagia
  - Neuropathies
- Physical exam:
  - Head and neck ± fiber-optic exam
  - Neurologic exam including cranial nerves
- Laboratories:
  - CBC, BUN, Cr, LFTs, alkaline phosphatase, and LDH
- Imaging:
  - MRI of the primary site and neck ± upper mediastinum
  - CT chest with contrast ± CT abdomen and pelvis or PET/CT as indicated
- Pathology:
- FNA or ultrasound/CT-guided biopsy for accessible lesions
- Ideal candidate for SBRT re-irradiation: ≥2 years from the initial course of RT and GTV <25 cc

Treatment Indications

- Early-stage head and neck cancers are definitively managed by local therapy, with single-modality surgical resection or external beam radiation therapy (EBRT) as the usual standard of care.
- Multimodal therapy, nearly always including EBRT combined with surgery, chemotherapy, or both, is frequently employed for locally or regionally advanced head and neck cancer.
- SBRT has been reported as a fractionated stereotactic boost for locally advanced nasopharyngeal cancers and oropharyngeal cancer and is also being evaluated for the treatment of early-stage laryngeal cancer.
- SBRT can be selectively used for small-volume recurrence or palliation.
- The combination of SBRT with concurrent targeted therapy or immunotherapy is under evaluation, but these combinations remain investigational.
- A few reports exist utilizing SBRT in the elderly or those unfit to undergo longer courses of EBRT or other definitive therapy.

Radiosurgical Technique

Simulation and Treatment Planning

- Thin-cut CT (1–1.5 mm) thickness recommended.
- GTV contoured from fusion of diagnostic imaging, merged in the area of interest to the planning CT.
- CTV margins may range from 0 to 10 mm depending on the clinical scenario:
  - Generally, no margin is required for microscopic extension.
  - Margins up to 5–10 mm may be considered if tumor infiltration into surrounding tissues is poorly delineated.

- PTV = CTV + 1–5 mm (dependent upon available center-specific image guidance and site-specific motion considerations).
- State-of-the-art tracking localization or frequent IGRT is recommended to reduce setup uncertainty and margins.
- Goal should be for low-dose to proximal OARs, achieved by use of an increased number of beams and angles, as well as minimization of margins.
- Phantom-based QA on all treatment plans prior to delivery.

Dose Prescription

- Dose and fractionation outside of the range of conventional fractionation for head and neck cancer (1.8–2.0 Gy/fraction/day) are not clearly defined in terms of alterations in safety profile or gains in efficacy.
- Planning should be determined with a high level of attention to potential adjacent normal tissue toxicity.
- For re-irradiation, the most commonly reported dose range is 30–50 Gy over 5 fractions.
- Ideally prescribe to ≥80% isodose line (IDL), ≥95% PTV coverage with prescription dose; depending on the characteristics of treatment planning system, 50–60% IDL is acceptable only if high-dose heterogeneity and falloff are thoroughly reviewed for safety.
- Composite planning should be employed in cases of re-irradiation, with appropriate BED conversion for dose summation.

Dose Limitations

- Ling et al. (2016): SBRT for re-irradiation of larynx or hypopharynx carcinoma may result in increased toxicity compared to SBRT to other sites. According to a dose-response model created to predict for severe late laryngeal toxicity, risk with D5cc of 5 Gy is 5.8%. This risk rises to 11.4% with a D5cc of 20 Gy and 25.3% with a D5cc of 40 Gy.

- Iqbal et al. (2021): Systemic review with 35–40 Gy in 5-fraction SBRT re-irradiation suggested constraints: Dmax carotid artery 32.5 Gy, optic chiasm/nerves 25 Gy; Dmean larynx 15 Gy, cochlea 15 Gy, retina 15 Gy, temporal tips 5 Gy.
- Grimm et al. (2021): Per HyTEC data pooling analysis, potential strategies to reduce carotid blowout or bleeding events in SBRT re-irradiation include treatment on nonconsecutive days, limiting circumferential irradiation if possible, as well as keeping D0.5cc <20 Gy and the re-irradiated major vessel volume exceeding 20–30 Gy as low as possible for 5-fraction SBRT.

Dose Delivery

- Dose often delivered in fractions given every other day; consecutive daily treatments should warrant additional caution.
- Setup may be isocentric or non-isocentric depending upon SBRT delivery system.
- Verification by kV XR or CBCT, aligned to visualized tumor or surrogate markers of position.
- Flexion of the cervical neck can result in interfractional variability of setup of a few millimeters.
- Intrafractional tumor motion may be as much as several millimeters in areas affected by jaw opening or laryngeal/swallowing motions.

Toxicities and Management

- Common acute toxicities (<6 weeks):
  - Fatigue:
    - Generally early-onset and self-limiting.

- Dermatitis::
  - Entrance and exit doses can be reduced with increased numbers of beams to minimize radiation dermatitis.
  - Mild-to-moderate: skin reaction treated with supportive care, including topical moisturizers, analgesics, low-dose steroids, and antimicrobial salves.
- Mucositis:
  - Critical to minimize target volumes to reduce pain and dysphagia related to this toxicity.
  - Treated with topical preparations including lidocaine-based solutions and pain medications.
  - Nutritional status should be carefully monitored.
- Severe late toxicities (>6 weeks):

  - Brachial plexopathy:
    - May present with neuropathic pain or with motor/sensory changes in the upper extremities.
    - MRI of brachial plexus and upper spine may be diagnostic and rule out tumor recurrence.
    - Limited treatment options include supportive care and occupational therapy.
  - Skin or soft-tissue necrosis::
    - For persistent nonhealing lesions, consider hyperbaric oxygen therapy and tocopherol pharmacotherapy.
  - Esophageal stricture or fistula:
    - Can occur after treatment of hypopharyngeal or cervical esophageal inlet.
    - More possible in the re-irradiation setting.
    - Treatment options include dilation or stent placement.
  - Vasculopathy:
    - Vascular erosion may lead to limited hemoptysis or massive hemorrhage and death (especially seen in re-irradiation setting).
    - Consider prophylactic stent placement.

- Osteoradionecrosis:
  - May occur in the jaw, skull base, or spine.
  - Worsened by infectious complications and in proximity to vascular structures, may raise the risk of hemorrhage.
- Brain necrosis:
  - Highest risk within areas of high cumulative dose.
  - May require neurosurgical intervention and potentially fatal.

Recommended Follow-Up

- CT or PET/CT every 3–4 months × 3 years, every 6 months × 2 years, every 12 months thereafter for routine follow-up.
- Neurologic/vascular status should be carefully followed; symptoms of headache, dizziness, or TIA should be investigated immediately.
- Infectious complications of the soft tissue or bone must be vigorously addressed due to high potential for osteoradionecrosis, soft-tissue necrosis, and/or vascular exposure and blowout.

Evidence

Boost/Recurrence for Nasopharyngeal Carcinoma

- Yau et al. (2004): 52 patients, EBRT 66 Gy with either 20 Gy intracavitary ^{192}Ir HDR (median 4–10 Gy × 2–5 fx, twice weekly) or SBRT (7.5 Gy × 2 fx or 2.5 Gy × 8 fx) boost. Patients were selected due to suspicion for persistent localized disease at several weeks after EBRT completion. Three-year LC in the no-boost, brachytherapy, and SBRT groups were 43, 71, and 82%.

- Chen et al. (2006): 64 patients, EBRT 64–68 Gy followed by 12–15 Gy SBRT boost, 60% with concurrent cisplatin. Three-year LC 93% and OS 84%. Three patients with large primary tumors had vascular bleeding resulting in death.
- Wu et al. (2007): SBRT to 90 patients with either persistent (6 Gy × 3 fx) or recurrent (8 Gy × 6 fx) NPC. Three-year LC and DSS were 89.4% and 80.7% for persistence, and 75.1% and 45.9% for recurrence. Seventeen (19%) patients developed severe late complications: six with mucosal necrosis, six with brain stem necrosis, six with temporal lobe necrosis, and two with fatal hemorrhage.
- Hara et al. (2008): 82 patients, EBRT 66 Gy followed by single-fraction median 11 Gy (range 7–15 Gy) SBRT boost. Eighty-five percent with concurrent cisplatin. Five-year LC 98% and OS 69%. Four patients had acute facial numbness. Late toxicities included three patients with retinopathy, one with carotid aneurysm, and ten cases of temporal lobe necrosis especially in those with T4 tumors.
- Yamazaki et al. (2014): 25 patients, EBRT median 50 Gy followed by SBRT boost median 15 Gy in 3 fx (range 12–35 Gy in 1–5 fx). Five-year LC 71% and OS 70%. PTV $\leq$20 cm^3 with better PFS (92%) and OS (100%).

Boost for Oropharyngeal Carcinoma

- Al-Mamgani et al. (2012): 51 patients, IMRT 46 Gy followed by ^{192}Ir PDR (mean 22 Gy, 8 fx per day $\geq$3 h intervals) or Cyberknife SBRT boost (5.5 Gy × 3). Those with node-positive disease underwent neck dissection. Three-year LC, DFS, and OS were 70%, 66%, and 54%. Acute grade 3 toxicities included dysphagia (45%), mucositis (25%), and dermatitis (16%).

Late grade 3 toxicities included dysphagia (4%) with one patient requiring a feeding tube at 2 years after treatment and xerostomia (4%).

- Baker et al. (2019): 195 patients, IMRT 46 Gy followed by SBRT boost (5.5 Gy × 3). Five-year DSS 85% and OS 67%. Late grade ≥3 toxicity 28% including soft-tissue necrosis (18%), dysphagia (12%), and osteoradionecrosis (9%).

Postoperative

- Vargo et al. (2014b): 28 patients re-irradiated with SBRT 40–44 Gy in 5 fractions over 1–2 weeks with concurrent cetuximab following salvage surgery with high-risk features (positive surgical margins or extra-nodal extension). One-year LRC and OS 51% and 64%. Acute and late grade ≥3 toxicity 0 and 8%.
- Biau et al. (2020): STEREO POSTOP GORTEC 2017-03 Phase II ongoing multicenter study, first prospective trial evaluating postoperative, hypofractionated SBRT (36 Gy in 6 fractions) in oropharyngeal and oral cavity cancers with high risk margins.

Laryngeal Carcinoma

- Schwartz et al. (2017): Phase I SBRT trial for Tis-T2N0 glottic laryngeal cancer. Twenty patients treated with incrementally shorter schedules: 50 Gy in 15 fx, 45 Gy in 10 fx, and finally 42.5 Gy in 5 fx. SBRT was delivered on a Cyberknife machine every other day. Patients received dexamethasone 4 mg an hour prior to each radiation treatment starting with the second cohort. Protocol-defined dose-limiting toxicities were not observed. Acute toxicities across all cohorts were limited to grade 1 or 2 and late toxicities. The second cohort had one patient experience grade 3 dysphagia and one patient experience grade 4 laryngeal edema. The first and third cohorts did not experience any grade 3 or greater late toxicity.

Locoregionally Recurrent Head and Neck Cancer (Re-irradiation)

- Heron et al. (2009): Phase I dose escalation study of re-irradiation for recurrent unresectable head and neck squamous cell carcinoma (HNSCC). Thirty-one patients with oropharynx, oral cavity, larynx, nasopharynx, and unknown primary cancers were treated in five tiers ranging from 25 to 44 Gy in 5 fractions over 2 weeks. Median prior dose of EBRT was 64.7 Gy, and 56% had received prior concurrent chemoradiation. Twenty-five patients were evaluable for toxicity, in whom no grade 3 complications were reported; the maximally tolerated dose was not reached.
- Cengiz et al. (2011): 46 patients with nasopharynx, oral cavity, paranasal sinus, larynx, and hypopharynx cancers re-irradiated with SBRT to doses from 18 to 45 Gy over 1–5 fractions. One-year local control and survival rates were 84 and 46%. Eight patients had carotid artery blowout and died. This occurred only in patients receiving 100% of the dose to the carotid artery and in whom tumor surrounded the carotid artery by at least 180°.
- Vargo et al. (2012): 150 patients' prospectively reported quality-of-life outcomes following SBRT to a dose of 40–50 Gy in 5 fractions with or without cetuximab for locally recurrent, previously irradiated head and neck cancers. These patients had previously received >40 Gy. After a median follow-up of 6 months (range 1–42), patient-reported quality of life progressively improved after an initial 1-month decline post-re-irradiation. Domains in swallowing, speech, saliva, activity, and

recreation showed statistical improvement compared to baseline.

- Kress et al. (2015): 85 patients re-irradiated with SBRT at a median 32 months from the first course of RT. Twenty-nine percent underwent surgical resection before SBRT. Seventy percent with induction, concurrent, or adjuvant chemotherapy or EGFR targeted therapy. Two-year LRC and OS 28% and 24%. Five patients (6%) with grade ≥3 late toxicity.
- Vargo et al. (2018): 414 patients from 8 institutions with unresectable recurrent or second primary HNSCC previously irradiated to ≥40 Gy. Comparable OS when ≥35 Gy SBRT delivered to small tumors GTV <25 cc.
- Lee et al. (2020): Meta-analysis of 10 studies with a total of 575 patients who underwent SBRT re-irradiation with a median dose range of 24–44 Gy in 3–6 fractions found pooled 2-year local control to be 47.3% and 2-year OS to be 30%. Pooled rate of clinical response was 61.7%, and complete response was 31.3%. 9.6% of patients experienced grade 3 or greater toxicity, and 4.6% experienced grade 5 toxicity.

SBRT with Concurrent Systemic Therapy

- Unger et al. (2010): 65 patients re-irradiated with SBRT, of whom 33 received concurrent chemotherapy or cetuximab. Patients receiving <30 Gy over 5 fractions had a 29% response rate versus 69% for higher doses. Two-year LRC and OS rates were 30% and 41%. Nineteen patients experienced grade 1–3 toxicity, and 7 experienced severe toxicity including one death. Chemotherapy did not improve outcomes on multivariable analysis, attributable to the small sample size and heterogeneity of agents used.
- Lartigau et al. (2013): Multi-institutional phase II study, 60 patients with inoperable recurrence or new primary HNSCC (size ≤65 mm) re-irradiated with

SBRT and cetuximab. Eighty percent were oropharyngeal tumors. Forty-eight percent had prior chemotherapy, and 93% had more than 20 pack-year smoking history. The mean time between prior RT and SBRT was 38 months. The SBRT dose was 36 Gy in 6 fractions in 11–12 days, prescribed at the 85% IDL, given with 1 loading and 4 concurrent cycles of concurrent cetuximab. If the spinal cord had received ≥45 Gy previously, the maximum allowed point dose was ≤6 Gy. Tumors with skin infiltration or invading more than 1/3 of the carotid artery were "avoided." Among 56 patients who completed SBRT-cetuximab with a follow-up of 11.4 months, 18 had grade 3 toxicities including mucositis, dysphagia, fistula, induration, and fibrosis. One patient died from hemorrhage and malnutrition. At 3 months, response and disease control rates were 58.4% and 91.7%. Median survival was 11.8 months, median progression-free survival was 7.1 months, and 1-year overall survival was 47.5%. Per intention to treat analysis, 33% had progressive disease.

■ Vargo et al. (2015): Phase II 50 patients with locally recurrent, unresectable, HNSCC previously irradiated to >60 Gy treated with cetuximab and SBRT re-irradiation. Forty-two percent oropharyngeal and 29% oral cavity tumors. Median time to re-irradiation was 18 months. Loading dose of cetuximab 400 mg/m², IV infusion, over 120 min on day 7, followed by 250 mg/m² on days 0 and 8 of SBRT. Tumors <25 cm³ were treated with SBRT 40 Gy in 5 fractions every other day while those ≥25 cm³ received 44 Gy. The 1-year locoregional PFS was 37%, 1-year distant PFS was 33%, and median OS was 10 months with a 1-year OS of 40%. Six percent of patients experienced acute grade 3 toxicity, and 6% experienced late grade 3 toxicity. There was no grade 4 toxicities. At the time of last quality of life survey, 62% of patients reported stable or improved quality of life over the last week.

- Wong et al. (2020): RTOG 3507, KEYSTROKE, is a phase II trial currently evaluating the safety of SBRT with or without pembrolizumab in the re-irradiation of head and neck cancer.
- McBride et al. (2021): Single-center randomized phase II trial of nivolumab ± SBRT (9 Gy × 3 fx to 1 lesion) in metastatic HNSCC. Grade 3–5 toxicities similar (13.3% vs. 9.7%). No difference in ORR of nonirradiated lesions (35% vs. 29%) and thus no evidence of an abscopal effect.

SBRT for Elderly or Medically Unfit

- Vargo et al. (2014a): Retrospective study of SBRT used as a primary treatment for elderly patients with medically inoperable head and neck cancers. Twelve patients with a median age of 88 years received primarily 44 Gy in 5 fractions every other day. Three patients received concurrent cetuximab, three patients had initial surgery and were treated for local recurrence, and two patients had received incomplete prior EBRT. One-year LC, PFS, and OS were 69%, 69%, and 64%. One acute grade 3 dysphagia and one late grade 3 mucositis without any grade 4 or 5 toxicities.
- Gogineni et al. (2020): Prospective study of 66 patients deemed unable to tolerate conventional definitive treatment who received SBRT to the GTV to a dose of 35–40 Gy in 5 fractions delivered biweekly. Median age was 80 years, and 48% of patients also received systemic therapy. One-year LC 73% and OS 64%. Two acute grade 3 toxicities and no grade 4 or 5 toxicities.

References

Al-Mamgani A, Tans L, Teguh DN, van Rooij P, Zwijnenburg EM, Levendag PC. Stereotactic body radiotherapy: a promising treatment option for the boost of oropharyngeal cancers not suitable for brachytherapy: a single-institutional experience. Int J Radiat Oncol Biol Phys. 2012;82(4):1494–500.

Baker S, Verduijn GM, Petit S, Sewnaik A, Mast H, Koljenović S, Nuyttens JJ, Heemsbergen WD. Long-term outcomes following stereotactic body radiotherapy boost for oropharyngeal squamous cell carcinoma. Acta Oncol. 2019;58(6):926–33.

Biau J, Thivat E, Millardet C, Saroul N, Pham-Dang N, Molnar I, Pereira B, Durando X, Bourhis J, Lapeyre M. A multicenter prospective phase II study of postoperative hypofractionated stereotactic body radiotherapy (SBRT) in the treatment of early-stage oropharyngeal and oral cavity cancers with high risk margins: the STEREO POSTOP GORTEC 2017-03 trial. BMC Cancer. 2020;20(1):730.

Cengiz M, Ozyigit G, Yazici G, Dogan A, Yildiz F, et al. Salvage reirradiation with stereotactic body radiotherapy for locally recurrent head-and-neck tumors. Int J Radiat Oncol Biol Phys. 2011;81:104–9.

Chen HH, Tsai ST, Wang MS, Wu YH, Hsueh WT, et al. Experience in fractionated stereotactic body radiation therapy boost for newly diagnosed nasopharyngeal carcinoma. Int J Radiat Oncol Biol Phys. 2006;66:1408–14.

Gogineni E, Rana Z, Vempati P, Karten J, Sharma A, Taylor P, Pereira L, Frank D, Paul D, Seetharamu N, Ghaly M. Stereotactic body radiotherapy as primary treatment for elderly and medically inoperable patients with head and neck cancer. Head Neck. 2020;42(10):2880–6.

Grimm J, Marks LB, Jackson A, Kavanagh BD, Xue J, Yorke E. High dose per fraction, Hypofractionated Treatment Effects in the Clinic (HyTEC): an overview. Int J Radiat Oncol Biol Phys. 2021;110(1):1–10.

Hara W, Loo BW Jr, Goffinet DR, Chang SD, Adler JR, et al. Excellent local control with stereotactic radiotherapy boost after external beam radiotherapy in patients with nasopharyngeal carcinoma. Int J Radiat Oncol Biol Phys. 2008;71:393–400.

Heron DE, Ferris RL, Karamouzis M, Andrade RS, Deeb EL, et al. Stereotactic body radiotherapy for recurrent squamous cell carcinoma of the head and neck: results of a phase I dose-escalation trial. Int J Radiat Oncol Biol Phys. 2009;75:1493–500.

Iqbal MS, West N, Richmond N, Kovarik J, Gray I, Willis N, Morgan D, Yazici G, Cengiz M, Paleri V, Kelly C. A systematic review and practical considerations of stereotactic body radiotherapy in the treatment of head and neck cancer. Br J Radiol. 2021;94(1117):20200332.

Kress MA, Sen N, Unger KR, Lominska CE, Deeken JF, Davidson BJ, Newkirk KA, Hwang J, Harter KW. Safety and efficacy of hypofractionated stereotactic body reirradiation in head and neck cancer: long-term follow-up of a large series. Head Neck. 2015;37(10):1403–9.

Lartigau EF, Tresch E, Thariat J, Graff P, Coche-Dequeant B, et al. Multi institutional phase II study of concomitant stereotactic reirradiation and cetuximab for recurrent head and neck cancer. Radiother Oncol. 2013;109:281–5.

Lee J, Kim WC, Yoon WS, Koom WS, Rim CH. Reirradiation using stereotactic body radiotherapy in the management of recurrent or second primary head and neck cancer: a meta-analysis and systematic review. Oral Oncol. 2020;107:104757.

Ling DC, Vargo JA, Ferris RL, Ohr J, Clump DA, Yau WY, Duvvuri U, Kim S, Johnson JT, Bauman JE, Branstetter BF. Risk of severe toxicity according to site of recurrence in patients treated with stereotactic body radiation therapy for recurrent head and neck cancer. Int J Radiat Oncol Biol Phys. 2016;95(3):973–80.

McBride S, Sherman E, Tsai CJ, Baxi S, Aghalar J, Eng J, Zhi WI, McFarland D, Michel LS, Young R, Lefkowitz R. Randomized phase II trial of nivolumab with stereotactic body radiotherapy versus nivolumab alone in metastatic head and neck squamous cell carcinoma. J Clin Oncol. 2021;39(1):30–7.

Schwartz DL, Sosa A, Chun SG, Ding C, Xie XJ, Nedzi LA, Timmerman RD, Sumer BD. SBRT for early-stage glottic larynx cancer—Initial clinical outcomes from a phase I clinical trial. PloS one. 2017;12(3):e0172055.

Unger KR, Lominska CE, Deeken JF, Davidson BJ, Newkirk KA, et al. Fractionated stereotactic radiosurgery for reirradiation of head-and-neck cancer. Int J Radiat Oncol Biol Phys. 2010;77:1411–9.

Vargo JA, Heron DE, Ferris RL, Rwigema JC, Wegner RE, Kalash R, Ohr J, Kubicek GJ, Burton S. Prospective evaluation of patient-reported quality-of-life outcomes following SBRT ± cetuximab for locally-recurrent, previously-irradiated head and neck cancer. Radiother Oncol. 2012;104(1):91–5.

Vargo JA, Ferris RL, Clump DA, Heron DE. Stereotactic body radiotherapy as primary treatment for elderly patients with medically inoperable head and neck cancer. Front Oncol. 2014a;4:214.

Vargo JA, Ferris RL, Ohr J, Clump DA, Davis KS, Duvvuri U, Kim S, Johnson JT, Bauman JE, Gibson MK, Branstetter BF. A prospective phase 2 trial of reirradiation with stereotactic body radiation therapy plus cetuximab in patients with previously irradiated recurrent squamous cell carcinoma of the head and neck. Int J Radiat Oncol Biol Phys. 2015;91(3):480–8.

Vargo JA, Kubicek GJ, Ferris RL, Duvvuri U, Johnson JT, Ohr J, Clump DA, Burton S, Heron DE. Adjuvant stereotactic body radiotherapy ± cetuximab following salvage surgery in previously irradiated head and neck cancer. Laryngoscope. 2014b;124(7):1579–84.

Vargo JA, Ward MC, Caudell JJ, Riaz N, Dunlap NE, Isrow D, Zakem SJ, Dault J, Awan MJ, Higgins KA, Hassanadeh C. A multi-institutional comparison of SBRT and IMRT for definitive reir-radiation of recurrent or second primary head and neck cancer. Int J Radiat Oncol Biol Phys. 2018;100(3):595–605.

Wong S, Torres-Saavedra P, Le QT, Chung C, Jang S, Huq MS, Jordan R, Clump DA, Blakaj DM, Straza MW, Koyfman S. Safety of reRT with SBRT plus concurrent and adjuvant pembrolizumab in patients with recurrent or new second primary head and neck squamous cell cancer in a previously irradiated field: RTOG 3507 foundation (KEYSTROKE). Int J Radiat Oncol Biol Phys. 2020;106(5):1224–5.

Wu SX, Chua DT, Deng ML, Zhao C, Li FY, et al. Outcome of frac-tionated stereotactic radiotherapy for 90 patients with locally persistent and recurrent nasopharyngeal carcinoma. Int J Radiat Oncol Biol Phys. 2007;69:761–9.

Yamazaki H, Ogita M, Himei K, Nakamura S, Yoshida K, Kotsuma T, Yamada Y, Fujiwara M, Baek S, Yoshioka Y. Hypofractionated stereotactic radiotherapy using CyberKnife as a boost treatment for head and neck cancer, a multi-institutional survey: impact of planning target volume. Anticancer Res. 2014;34(10):5755–9.

Yau TK, Sze WM, Lee WM, Yeung MW, Leung KC, et al. Effectiveness of brachytherapy and fractionated stereotactic radiotherapy boost for persistent nasopharyngeal carcinoma. Head Neck. 2004;26:1024–30.

Chapter 6
Lung

Katelyn Hasse and Jason W. Chan

Pearls

- Lung cancer incidence and mortality are ~225 k and 160 k per year: #1 in cancer deaths in the USA, more than breast, prostate, and colorectal combined.
- NSCLC death rates dropped by 5% annually from 2014 to 2018, and 2-year OS improved by 5–6% for every stage of diagnosis since 2009.
- Lobectomy is the standard of care for early-stage NSCLC though sublobar resections can be considered in select cases.
- SBRT is the standard of care for medically inoperable T1-2N0 NSCLC though it can be considered for select patients with tumors >5 cm.
- SBRT results in superior LC and possibly OS compared to conventionally fractionated EBRT for early-stage NSCLC.

K. Hasse · J. W. Chan (✉)
Department of Radiation Oncology, University of California, San Francisco, San Francisco, CA, USA
e-mail: katelyn.hasse@ucsf.edu; jason.w.chan@ucsf.edu

© The Author(s), under exclusive license to Springer Nature Switzerland AG 2023
R. A. Sethi et al. (eds.), *Handbook of Evidence-Based Stereotactic Radiosurgery and Stereotactic Body Radiotherapy*, https://doi.org/10.1007/978-3-031-33156-5_6

137

- Five-year local control for BED_{10} ≥100 is over 90%.
- SBRT for operable candidates is best considered on clinical trial, and involvement of multidisciplinary team is always recommended.

Workup

- H&P, including performance status, weight loss, and smoking status.
- Review of symptoms:
  - Most early-stage NSCLCs are asymptomatic.
  - More advanced presentations include cough, dyspnea, hemoptysis, post-obstructive pneumonia, pleural effusion, pain, hoarseness (left recurrent laryngeal nerve), SVC syndrome, clubbing, superior sulcus (Pancoast) tumor triad of shoulder pain, brachial plexopathy, and Horner's syndrome.
- Laboratories:
  - CBC, BUN, Cr, LFTs, alkaline phosphatase, and LDH.
- Imaging:
  - Chest, abdomen, and pelvis staging CT with contrast (r/o liver and adrenal metastases).
  - PET/CT (>90% negative predictive value for nodal involvement, but low sensitivity for adenocarcinoma in situ (AIS); unclear association of max SUV with SBRT outcomes).
  - MRI brain for stage ≥ II (consider for stage IB) and/or if neurologic symptoms on presentation.
  - MRI thoracic inlet for superior sulcus tumors for assessment of brachial plexus and vertebral involvement.
- Pathology:
  - CT-guided biopsy of peripheral N0 lesions.

- Mediastinoscopy or bronchoscopic biopsy for central tumors and/or N+ disease.
- Thoracentesis for pleural effusions.
- Biomarker testing for EGFR mutations, ALK/ROS1/RET gene rearrangements, BRAF/KRAS point mutations, METex14 skipping variants, NTRK gene fusions, PD-L1 expression.
- Pulmonary function testing for presurgical and preradiotherapy evaluation:
  - Medically inoperable for lobectomy is generally FEV1 <40% or <1.2 L, DLCO ≤50%, FVC <70% but less restrictive if wedge/segmentectomy is planned.

Treatment Indications

- SBRT is the standard of care of T1-2N0 NSCLC and SCLC in medically inoperable patients or when surgical resection is not pursued.
- Most established SBRT criteria include N0 patients with <5 cm, peripherally located tumors, but tumors may be more cautiously treated with expanded criteria of larger size (<7 cm), central location, multiple synchronous lesions, and chest wall invasion (T3N0) with historically inferior results.
- SBRT has a developing role as a boost following definitive chemoradiation in the management of locally advanced NSCLC, for re-irradiation of locally recurrent disease, and for treatment of intrathoracic oligometastases from various primary histologies (commonly stage IV NSCLC, sarcoma, renal cell carcinoma, thyroid, or colorectal cancer) (Table 6.1).

TABLE 6.1 Treatment recommendations for NSCLC and pulmonary oligometastases

Presentation	Resectability	Recommended treatment
T1-2N0	Operable	Lobectomy (consider segmentectomy for ≤2 cm) or SBRT
	Inoperable	SBRT (may consider RFA/cryotherapy)
II (T2bN0, T1-2N1, T3N0)	Operable	Surgery → chemo (>4 cm)
	Inoperable	ChemoRT → immunotherapy or hypofx EBRT → ± chemo
IIIA	Operable	ChemoRT → restage → surgery → chemo or chemo → restage → surgery → chemo ± RT
	Inoperable	ChemoRT → immunotherapy
IIIB	Inoperable	ChemoRT → immunotherapy
Recurrent	Operable	EBRT/SBRT/resection for limited local recurrence → systemic therapy
	Inoperable	EBRT/SBRT/RFA/cryo for limited recurrence → systemic therapy
Pulmonary oligometastases	Operable	Lobectomy/wedge resection or SBRT or hypofractionated EBRT (for larger lesions, >5 cm) → systemic therapy
	Inoperable	SBRT, RFA, cryo, or hypofx EBRT (preferred for larger lesions, >5 cm) → systemic therapy

Radiosurgical Technique

Simulation and Treatment Planning

■ Tumor motion may be 2–3 cm in peri-diaphragmatic regions of the lower lung. Motion management strategies include respiratory gating, coaching with audiovisual feedback, breath-hold techniques, abdominal compression, and intrafraction tumor tracking real-time imaging techniques with dynamic beam and/or couch compensation.

■ Thin-cut CT (≤1.5 mm) thickness recommended. 4D CT or maximal inspiratory and expiratory phase CTs or slow CT recommended to assess target and critical structure internal motion. Free-breathing helical or mean intensity projection CT should be used for dose calculation.

■ iGTV contoured from maximum intensity projection (MIP) generated from 4D CT. MIP should be used judiciously in tumors adjacent to diaphragm or chest wall, with additional imaging as needed to fully discriminate the target from surrounding normal tissue with similar CT tissue density.

■ GTV/iGTV = tumor visible on CT lung window.

■ CTV/ITV = GTV/iGTV + 0–10 mm (in RTOG protocols, GTV and CTV have been considered identical on CT planning with zero expansion margin added).

■ PTV = CTV/ITV + 3–10 mm (dependent upon available center-specific IGRT and motion management capabilities). Current RTOG guidelines are:

　◆ Non-4D CT planning, PTV = GTV + 5 mm axial and 10 mm longitudinal anisotropic margins.

　◆ 4D CT planning, PTV = ITV + 5 mm isotropic margin.

■ Dose to proximal OARs attributed to compact intermediate dose region outside of the CTV/ITV region, generally reduced with increased beams and angles, as well as minimization of margins on target.

- Treatment planning guidelines (adapted from RTOG 0618):
  - V_{Rx} dose $\geq$ 95% PTV, V90 $\geq$ 99% PTV.
  - High-dose region ($\geq$105% Rx dose) should fall within the PTV.
  - Conformality index goal $\leq$1.2.
- Heterogeneity correction algorithms are recommended (anisotropic analytical algorithm, collapsed cone convolution, Monte Carlo, etc.). Pencil beam algorithms that overestimate dose in heterogeneous tissue are not recommended.
- Phantom-based QA on treatment plans.

Dose Prescription

- Dose and fractionation directed by adjacent normal tissue RT toxicity constraints with goal tumor BED_{10} >100. Adaptive dosimetry for histology-, volume-, location-, and context-based lesions (primary vs. metastatic) is under investigation.
- Current dose fractionation schema largely employs 1–5 fractions.
- Peripheral lung tumors:
  - *Common accepted schemas*: 25–34 Gy × 1 fraction, 18 Gy × 3 fractions, 12 Gy × 4 fractions, 10 Gy × 5 fractions.
- Central lung tumors:
  - *We recommend* 10 Gy × 5 fractions (BED_{10} dose limited to reduce toxicity of central structures: large airways, heart, esophagus, and spinal cord). See Fig. 6.1.
- Dose typically prescribed 60–90% IDL, with $\geq$95% PTV coverage by prescription dose.
- Composite planning should be employed in cases of regional lung re-irradiation with appropriate BED conversion for dose summation.

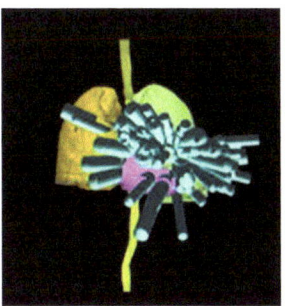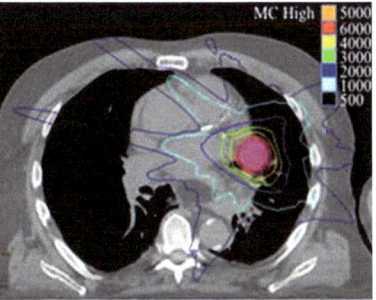

FIG. 6.1 SBRT planning for a central early-stage NSCLC. Beam distribution shown on 3D anatomy reconstruction (left) and dose distribution for 50 Gy given in 5 fractions (right)

Dose Limitations

- See Table 6.2, assuming no prior regional radiotherapy (TG 101, Benedict et al. 2010; RTOG 0618).

Dose Delivery

- Dose delivered in consecutive daily or every other day fractions as per NRG protocols.
- Setup may be isocentric or non-isocentric depending upon SBRT delivery system.
- Verification by kV XR or CBCT, aligned to visualized tumor or surrogate.
- Intrafraction dose delivery adjustment by motion management and IGRT systems as discussed above.

Toxicities and Management

- Common acute toxicities (<6 weeks):
  - Fatigue:
    - *Generally early-onset and* self-limiting.

TABLE 6.2 Recommended dose constraints for SBRT lung lesion target planning

Structure	Fractions	Constraints
Lung	1	V7 < 1500 cc
	3	V11.6 < 1500 cc
	5	V12.5 < 1500 cc
Central airway	1	V10.5 < 4 cc, Dmax 20.2 Gy
	3	V15 < 4 cc, Dmax 30 Gy
	5	V16.5 < 4 cc, Dmax 40 Gy
Chest wall	1	V22 < 1 cc, Dmax 30 Gy
	3	V28.8 < 1 cc, Dmax 36.9 Gy
	5	V35 < 1 cc, Dmax 43 Gy
Heart	1	V16 < 15 cc, Dmax 22 Gy
	3	V24 < 15 cc, Dmax 30 Gy
	5	V32 < 15 cc, Dmax 38 Gy
Esophagus	1	V11.9 < 5 cc, Dmax 15.4 Gy
	3	V17.7 < 5 cc, Dmax 25.2 Gy
	5	V19.5 < 5 cc, Dmax 35 Gy
Brachial plexus	1	V14 < 3 cc, Dmax 17.5 Gy
	3	V20.4 < 3 cc, Dmax 24 Gy
	5	V 27 < 3 cc, Dmax 30.5 Gy
Spinal cord	1	V10 < 0.35 cc, Dmax 14 Gy
	3	V18 < 0.35 cc, Dmax 21.9 Gy
	5	V23 < 0.35 cc, Dmax 30 Gy
Skin	1	V23 < 10 cc, Dmax 26 Gy
	3	V30 < 10 cc, Dmax 33 Gy
	5	V36.5 < 10 cc, Dmax 39.5 Gy

- *Sustained fatigue may* be related to cardiopulmonary dysfunction (CHF, CAD, COPD, etc.) and warrants further workup.
- Cough/dyspnea
  - *Low-grade cough common* secondary to RT-related intrapulmonary inflammation. Antitussive pharmacotherapy for mild symptoms.
  - *Severity of shortness* of breath may be related to baseline lung function and associated comorbidities. For patients with moderate-to-severe symptoms or significant baseline comorbidities (COPD, ILD, CHF, etc.), recommend follow-up with pulmonology and/or cardiology.
- Chest pain:
  - *May be related* to regional pleuritis and/or pericarditis and is generally self-limited.
  - *Analgesic pharmacotherapy recommended.*
- Pneumonitis:
  - *Associated with increased* dose volume (V20 < 10%), smoking history (current/former), age, prior use of steroids, and comorbidity index on multiple studies.
  - *Generally subacute onset* (>2 weeks), associated with cough, dyspnea, hypoxia, and fever.
  - *If symptomatic, treat* with prednisone (1 mg/kg/day) or 60 mg/day and trimethoprim/sulfamethoxazole for PCP prophylaxis. Symptomatic relief may be rapid, but slow steroid taper is critical for durable symptom resolution.
- Esophagitis:
  - *Increased risk with* treatment centrally located tumors and is generally self-limited to several weeks after treatment.
  - *Local or systemic* analgesic pharmacotherapy (lidocaine, NSAIDs, opioids) ± proton pump inhibitor based on the severity of symptoms.
- Dermatitis:

- *Chest wall entrance* and exit doses can be reduced with increased numbers of beams to minimize radiation dermatitis.
- *Mild-to-moderate* skin reaction treated with supportive care, including topical moisturizers, analgesics, low-dose steroids, and antimicrobial salves.
- Common late toxicities (>6 weeks):
  - Persistent cough/dyspnea:
    - *Recommend consultation with* pulmonary medicine for consideration of long-term bronchodilator and anti-inflammatory therapy.
  - Radiation pneumonitis:
    - *Most commonly observed* at ~6 weeks.
    - *As above, recommend* steroids with gradual taper for symptomatic patients.
  - Brachial plexopathy:
    - *Apical lung tumors* associated with greater risk of brachial plexus injury.
    - *May present with* neuropathic pain as seen in Lhermitte's syndrome or with motor/sensory changes in the upper extremities.
    - MRI of brachial plexus and upper spine may be diagnostic and rule out tumor recurrence.
    - *Limited treatment options* include supportive care and occupational therapy.
  - Chest wall pain and rib fracture:
    - *More common in* patients with peripheral lesions.
    - Supportive care indicated.
  - Radiation skin ulcer:
    - *For persistent nonhealing* skin lesions, consider hyperbaric oxygen therapy and tocopherol pharmacotherapy.
  - Esophageal stricture and tracheoesophageal fistula:
    - *Historically rare complication* observed with the treatment of mediastinal lymphadenopathy in locally advanced lung cancer.

■ *Even less likely* with SBRT, if airway and esophageal constraints maintained, with exception of re-irradiation setting.
■ Vasculopathy:
   ■ *Vascular erosion may* lead to limited hemoptysis or massive hemorrhage and death (seen in re-irradiation setting of central lesions).

Recommended Follow-Up

■ CT chest ± contrast every 3–6 months × 3 years, every 6 months × 2 years, every 12 months thereafter for routine follow-up. ^{18}F-FDG PET should not routinely be used for surveillance.
■ Assessment with RECIST criteria of limited utility due to a wide spectrum of evolving radiographic features following SBRT including diffuse and patchy GGO, consolidation, and/or fibrosis.
■ In general, radiographic changes include early inflammatory response (≤3 months) followed by resolution of FDG activity and late fibrosis (>6 months) in the area of treated lesion, which is often dynamic and may evolve over several years.
■ Persistent increase in size and density of treated tumor on interval CTs in the early posttreatment setting (<12 months) or new densities at later times (>12 months) should be considered suspicious for recurrence, with recommendation for increased frequency of CT, interval PET scan, and consideration of biopsy and/or surgical or radiotherapy salvage procedure.
■ Role of molecular imaging and circulating tumor markers is under investigation.

Evidence

SBRT vs. Conventional Fractionation

- SPACE (Nyman et al. 2016): Phase II 102 medically inoperable stage I NSCLC randomized to SBRT 66 Gy in 3 fractions (to isocenter, 45 Gy to PTV) vs. 3D-CRT 70 Gy in 35 fractions. Similar OS and PFS and less toxicity despite larger tumors in SBRT arm. 1-, 2-, and 3-year PFS 76%, 53%, and 42%; 19% pneumonitis; 8% esophagitis in SBRT arm.
- CHISEL/TROG 09/02 (Ball et al. 2019): Phase III 101 medically inoperable peripheral stage I NSCLC randomized to SBRT 54 Gy in 3 fractions or 48 Gy in 4 fractions vs. 3D-CRT 66 Gy in 33 fractions or 50 Gy in 20 fractions. SBRT resulted in superior 2-year LC (86% vs. 69%) and OS (77% vs. 59%) without increase in major toxicity.

SBRT in Medically Operable Patients

- RTOG 0618 (Timmerman et al. 2018): Phase II study 54 Gy in 3 fractions. 26 of 33 accrued patients were evaluable. Four-year LC, DFS, and OS were 96%, 57%, and 56%. Grade 3 adverse events in 8%.
- STARS-ROSEL (Chang et al. 2015): Pooled analysis of 58 patients with cT1-2a (<4 cm) operable NSCLC randomized to lobectomy and mediastinal lymph node dissection vs. SBRT. STARS and ROSEL both closed early due to slow accrual. Three-year OS 95% in SBRT group compared to 79% in surgery group and fewer grade 3–4 toxicities, 10% vs. 44%. Three-year RFS similar, 86% vs. 80%.
- SABRTooth (Franks et al. 2020): Phase III RCT between SBRT and surgery could not accrue in NHS

due to preexisting treatment preferences (41% for SBRT and 19% for surgery).

- RTOG 3502 (NCT01753414) ongoing randomized phase II trial of sublobar resection vs. SBRT for stage I operable NSCLC.
- STABLE-MATES (NCT02468024) ongoing randomized phase II trial of sublobar resection vs. SBRT for "high" surgical risk patients.
- VALOR (NCT02984761) ongoing randomized phase III trial of lobectomy or segmentectomy vs. SBRT in 3–5 fractions.

Pre-op SBRT

- MISSLE (Palma et al. 2019a, b): Phase II study of SBRT followed by lobectomy or sublobar resection after 10 weeks in 40 patients with operable T1-2N0 NSCLC. pCR lower than hypothesized at 60%. Two-year LC 100%, regional control 53%, and distant control 76%.
- Altorki et al. (2021): Phase II study of durvalumab q3w for 2 cycles ± SBRT 24 Gy in 3 fractions prior to surgical resection. 60 patients with stage I–IIIA NSCLC. Higher rates of major pathologic responses with SBRT 53% vs. 7%.

SBRT Fractionation Comparisons

- RTOG 0915 (Videtic et al. 2019): Phase II 34 Gy in 1 fraction vs. 48 Gy in 4 fractions. Grade ≥ 3 toxicities 2.6% vs. 11.1%. Five-year outcomes similar, LC 89 vs. 93% and OS 30 vs. 41%.
- Singh et al. (2019): Phase II 30 Gy in 1 fraction vs. 60 Gy in 3 fractions. Similar 2-year LC 95% vs. 97%. Grade 3 toxicities 16% vs. 12%.

SBRT for Central and Ultracentral Tumors

- Timmerman et al. (2006): Phase II 54 Gy in 3 fractions with heterogeneity corrections. Grade ≥ 3 toxicity higher for central tumors (17 vs. 46%) helped establish "no-fly zone" of 2 cm around proximal bronchial tree.
- Cheung et al. (2014): Phase II 60 Gy in 15 fractions. 80 patients with tumors <5 cm not involving mainstem bronchi. Two-year LC, regional control, distant control, and OS were 87%, 91%, 78%, and 69%. Grade ≥ 3 toxicities 40%. Grade 4 and 5 toxicities 6% and 1%.
- Bezjak et al. (2019): Phase I/II dose escalation for medically inoperable central lesions 2 cm from proximal bronchial tree or PTV touching mediastinal or pericardial pleura. Maximum tolerated dose was 12 Gy per fractions associated with 7.2% dose-limiting toxicities. Grade ≥ 3 toxicity 24% in 10.5–11 Gy per fraction cohort (52.5–55 Gy in 5 fractions) and 21% in 11.5–12 Gy cohort (57.5–60 Gy in 5 fractions). Few tumors were ultracentral or overlapping with central organs other than bronchi and vessels (e.g., esophagus).
- HILUS (Lindberg et al. 2021): Phase II 56 Gy in 8 fractions prescribed to 67% isodose for tumors ≤ 1 cm from mainstem bronchi and trachea. Two-year LC 83%. 22 of 65 patients with grade 3–5 toxicities including 10 treatment-related pulmonary deaths.

SBRT for Large Tumors >5 cm

- Verma et al. (2017): Multi-institutional retrospective study of SBRT for ≥ 5 cm NSCLC. 92 patients treated with median 50 Gy. Two-year LC, DFS, DM, and OS were 72%, 54%, 33%, and 46%. Grade ≥ 3 toxicity 5%. Grade ≥ 2 toxicities lower with QOD vs. QD treatments, 7% vs. 43%.
- McDermott et al. (2021): Retrospective study of NSCLC ≥ 5 cm mostly treated with 60 Gy in 8 fractions

(78%). LC at 1, 2, and 3 years 85%, 71%, and 57%. Out-of-field intrapulmonary progression in 24%. Grade ≥3 toxicities in two patients with dyspnea.

SBRT for Re-irradiation

- Viani et al. (2020): Meta-analysis of 20 studies and 625 lesions in 595 patients (86% primary lung cancer) who underwent re-irradiation with SBRT. 51% previously treated with conventional RT. Two-year LC 73% and OS 54%. Cumulative dose ≤145 Gy versus >145 Gy EQD2 associated with 3% vs. 15% of any grade ≥3 toxicity.
- Rulach et al. (2021): International Expert Survey on Re-RT for NSCLC. Cumulative lung dose constraints not agreed upon but suggestions included.

SBRT for Oligometastases

- Ashworth et al. (2014): Meta-analysis of 757 NSCLC patients with 1–5 synchronous or metachronous metastases treated with local consolidative therapy. In RPA, three risk groups were identified: low-risk, metachronous metastases (5-year OS 47.8%); synchronous metastases and N0 (5-year OS 36.2%); and high-risk, synchronous metastases and N1/N2 disease (5-year OS 13.8%).
- Gomez et al. (2016, 2019): Phase II multi-institutional study randomized 49 NSCLC patients with ≤3 metastases after first-line systemic therapy to local consolidative therapy ([chemo]radiotherapy or resection of all lesions) with or without subsequent maintenance treatment or to maintenance treatment/observation alone (MT/O). LCT prolonged PFS (median 23.1 vs. 14.2 months) and OS (median 41.2 months vs. 17.0 months). Adverse events similar between groups.

- Iyengar et al. (2018): Phase II single-institution study randomized 29 NSCLC patients to maintenance chemo alone vs. SBRT followed by maintenance chemo for patients with oligometastatic NSCLC (primary and ≤ 5 metastases) after induction chemo. EGFR and ALK-driven NSCLC were excluded. Trial stopped early after interim analysis found PFS improvement in SBRT arm median 9.7 months vs. 3.5 months for four (29%) SBRT patients with grade 3 toxicities though no significant difference in rates of toxicities.
- SABR-COMET (Palma et al. 2019a, b, 2020): Phase II multi-institutional trial randomized 99 patients to the standard of care $\pm$ SABR, mostly 1–3 metastases of various tumor types, 18% lung primary, and 53% metastases located in lung. SABR arm had improved 5-year PFS (median NR vs. 17.3%) and OS (median 42.3% vs. 17.7%). More toxicities in SABR arm including 3 (4.5%) treatment-related deaths vs. none in control arm. Relatively low LC (51%) for lung lesions using RECIST version 1.1.

Technique

Dose Prescription

- ICRU-91 (de Jong et al. 2020): Minimum dose (D98%) BED_{10} of GTV/ITV 150 Gy and PTV 100 Gy. Maximum dose (D2%) in the range of 60–70 Gy.

Treatment Planning

- Desai et al. (2021): 102 SBRT VMAT plans. 32 plans with R50% and/or D2cm metrics higher than recommended tolerances in RTOG 0813 and 0915 were replanned with novel shell structures and constraints.

R50% violations can be rectified with a dose constraint to a novel shell structure ("OptiForR50"). Violations in D2cm can be rectified by using constraints on a 0.5 cm thick shell structure with inner surface 2 cm from the PTV surface.

Motion Management

■ Caillet et al. (2017): IGRT and motion management during lung SBRT delivery. Review of IGRT and motion management techniques available in radiation therapy. Clinical benefit of motion management is hard to interpret due to small cohorts, different treatment strategies, and lack of randomized trials. MRI-guided treatment may provide paradigm shift.

■ Yang et al. (2017): Target margin design with real-time tumor tracking. Retrospective analysis of 22 CyberKnife XSight Lung Tracking Patients. Total tracking errors were <4 mm in S-I, L-R, and A-P directions. With 4 mm global margin, 95% coverage in S-I direction and 100% coverage in L-R and A-P directions were obtained.

■ Sarudis et al. (2017): Analysis of lung tumor motion using 4D CT for 126 lung SBRT patients. Tumor motion was greatest in the S-I direction (average of 7 mm, maximum of 53 mm), specifically for middle and lower lobes of the lungs. A-P and L-R motion showed no correlation with location. Tumor size has no correlation with motion amplitude in any direction.

■ Brandner et al. (2017): A review from NRG oncology on motion management strategies and technical issues for thoracic SBRT. Found only 40% of lung tumors move more than 5 mm, with 12% moving more than 10 mm. Extent of tumor motion should be used to assign appropriate margins. End expiration phase is relatively stable, less affected by inconsistencies, and patients spend more time near end expiration than any other phase. If normal tissue tolerances (based on Quantec or relevant NRG/RTOG protocols or institutional criteria) are exceeded, or MLC interplay effects are a concern, consider motion-limiting techniques. Coaching is recommended for gating. Daily imaging guidance is required, and daily volumetric imaging is preferred. Heterogeneity corrections are required, and dose should be calculated with Monte Carlo or convolution/superposition algorithms.

- Fogliata and Cozzi (2017): Dose calculation accuracy for stereotactic treatment of lung lesions. Lung SBRT dose estimation and its accuracy are based on the difficulties of handling small fields and low density. Pencil beam algorithms are unsuitable, because they do not account for changes in electron transport, particularly changes in scatter from lateral heterogeneities. This results in erroneous dose estimation on the order of 20–30%. Convolution/superposition-type algorithms do account for lateral electron transport, but depending on the specific algorithm, errors can be on the order of 10%. Monte Carlo algorithms, which account for the chemical composition of the medium, are the current gold standard.

- Gandhidasan et al. (2021): Abdominal compression versus active breathing control (ABC). Retrospective analysis of 873 patients with 931 lesions treated with SBRT for either a primary lung cancer or oligometastases. No significant difference in local failure with motion management technique though central location may be associated with local failure with ABC (HR = 2.1, $p = 0.07$).

Follow-Up

- Trovo et al. (2010): Review of posttreatment CT scans of 68 patients (largely SBRT-treated early-stage NSCLC) from 6 weeks to 18 months. Early radiographic changes included diffuse and patchy consolidation and GGO, increased from 6 weeks (46%) to 6 months (79%). Late changes included consolidation, volume loss, and bronchiectasis with mass- and scar-like fibrosis in 88% of scans at >12 months.

- Bollneni et al. (2012): Review of 132 medically inoperable stage I NSCLC patients treated with 60 Gy in 3–8 fractions. Max SUV on PET/CT at 12 weeks ≥5.0 was associated with 2 years' LC of 80% vs. 98% for max SUV <5.0 ($p = 0.019$).
- Huang et al. (2013): Six imaging high-risk features (HRFs) were associated with local recurrence by reviewing serial imaging of 12 patients with local recurrences compared to 24 patients without local recurrences. PET/CT may be useful for ≤2 HRFs. For ≥3 HRFs, >90% sensitivity and specificity for local recurrence.

References

Altorki NK, McGraw TE, Borczuk AC, Saxena A, Port JL, Stiles BM, Lee BE, Sanfilippo NJ, Scheff RJ, Pua BB, Gruden JF. Neoadjuvant durvalumab with or without stereotactic body radiotherapy in patients with early-stage non-small-cell lung cancer: a single-center, randomized phase 2 trial. Lancet Oncol. 2021;22(6):824–35.

Ashworth AB, Senan S, Palma DA, Riquet M, Ahn YC, Ricardi U, Congedo MT, Gomez DR, Wright GM, Melloni G, Milano MT. An individual patient data metanalysis of outcomes and prognostic factors after treatment of oligometastatic non-small-cell lung cancer. Clin Lung Cancer. 2014;15(5):346–55.

Ball D, Mai GT, Vinod S, Babington S, Ruben J, Kron T, Chesson B, Herschtal A, Vanevski M, Rezo A, Elder C. Stereotactic ablative radiotherapy versus standard radiotherapy in stage 1 non-small-cell lung cancer (TROG 09.02 CHISEL): a phase 3, open-label, randomised controlled trial. The Lancet Oncology. 2019;20(4):494–503.

Bezjak A, Paulus R, Gaspar LE, Timmerman RD, Straube WL, Ryan WF, Garces YI, Pu AT, Singh AK, Videtic GM, McGarry

RC. Safety and efficacy of a five-fraction stereotactic body radio-therapy schedule for centrally located non–small-cell lung cancer: NRG oncology/RTOG 0813 trial. J Clin Oncol. 2019;37(15):1316.

Benedict SH, Yenice KM, Followill D, Galvin JM, Hinson W, Kavanagh B, Keall P, Lovelock M, Meeks S, Papiez L, Purdie T. Stereotactic body radiation therapy: the report of AAPM Task Group 101. Medical physics. 2010;37(8):4078–101.

Bollneni VR, Widder J, Pruim J, Langendijk JA, Wiegman EM. Residual ^{18}F-FDG-PET uptake 12 weeks after stereotactic ablative radiotherapy for stage I non-small-cell lung cancer pre-dicts local control. Int J Radiat Oncol Biol Phys. 2012;83(4):e551–5.

Brandner ED, Chetty IJ, Giaddui TG, Xiao Y, Huq MS. Motion man-agement strategies and technical issues associated with stereotac-tic body radiotherapy of thoracic and upper abdominal tumors: a review from NRG oncology. Med Phys. 2017;44(6):2595–612.

Caillet V, Booth JT, Keall P. IGRT and motion management during lung SBRT delivery. Phys Med. 2017;44:113–22.

Chang JY, Senan S, Paul MA, Mehran RJ, Louie AV, Balter P, Groen HJ, McRae SE, Widder J, Feng L, van den Borne BE. Stereotactic ablative radiotherapy versus lobectomy for operable stage I non-small-cell lung cancer: a pooled analysis of two randomized trials. Lancet Oncol. 2015;16(6):630–7.

Cheung P, Faria S, Ahmed S, Chabot P, Greenland J, Kurien E, Mohamed I, Wright JR, Hollenhorst H, de Metz C, Campbell H. Phase II study of accelerated hypofractionated three-dimensional conformal radiotherapy for stage T1-3 N0 M0 non–small cell lung cancer: NCIC CTG BR.25. J Natl Cancer Inst. 2014;106(8):dju164.

de Jong EE, Guckenberger M, Andratschke N, Dieckmann K, Hoogeman MS, Milder M, Møller DS, Nyeng TB, Tanadini-Lang S, Lartigau E, Lacornerie T. Variation in current prescrip-tion practice of stereotactic body radiotherapy for peripherally located early stage non-small cell lung cancer: recommendations for prescribing and recording according to the ACROP guideline and ICRU report 91. Radiother Oncol. 2020;142:217–23.

Desai D, Narayanasamy G, Bimali M, Cordrey I, Elasmar H, Srinivasan S, Johnson EL. Cleaning the dose falloff in lung SBRT plan. J Appl Clin Med Phys. 2021;22(1):100–8.

Fogliata A, Cozzi L. Dose calculation algorithm accuracy for small fields in non-homogeneous media: the lung SBRT case. Phys Med. 2017;44:157–62.

Franks KN, McParland L, Webster J, Baldwin DR, Sebag-Montefiore D, Evison M, Booton R, Faivre-Finn C, Naidu B, Ferguson J, Peedell C. SABRTooth: a randomized controlled feasibility study of stereotactic ablative radiotherapy (SABR) with surgery in patients with peripheral stage I nonsmall cell lung cancer considered to be at higher risk of complications from surgical resection. Eur Respir J. 2020;56(5):2000118.

Gandhidasan S, Woody NM, Stephans KL, Videtic GM. Does motion management technique for lung SBRT influence local control? A single institutional experience comparing abdominal compression to breath-hold technique. Pract Radiat Oncol. 2021;11(2):e180–5.

Gomez DR, Blumenschein GR Jr, Lee JJ, Hernandez M, Ye R, Camidge DR, Doebele RC, Skoulidis F, Gaspar LE, Gibbons DL, Karam JA. Local consolidative therapy versus maintenance therapy or observation for patients with oligometastatic non-small-cell lung cancer without progression after first-line systemic therapy: a multicenter, randomized, controlled, phase 2 study. Lancet Oncol. 2016;17(12):1672–82.

Gomez DR, Tang C, Zhang J, Blumenschein GR Jr, Hernandez M, Lee JJ, Ye R, Palma DA, Louie AV, Camidge DR, Doebele RC. Local consolidative therapy vs. maintenance therapy or observation for patients with oligometastatic non-small-cell lung cancer: long-term results of a multi-institutional, phase II, randomized study. J Clin Oncol. 2019;37(18):1558.

Huang K, Senthi S, Palma DA, Spoelstra FO, Warner A, Slotman BJ, Senan S. High-risk CT features for detection of local recurrence after stereotactic ablative radiotherapy for lung cancer. Radiother Oncol. 2013;109(1):51–7.

Iyengar P, Wardak Z, Gerber DE, Tumati V, Ahn C, Hughes RS, Dowell JE, Cheedella N, Nedzi L, Westover KD, Pulipparacharuvil S. Consolidative radiotherapy for limited metastatic non–small-cell lung cancer: a phase 2 randomized clinical trial. JAMA Oncol. 2018;4(1):e173501.

Lindberg K, Grozman V, Karlsson K, Lindberg S, Lax I, Wersäll P, Persson GF, Josipovic M, Khalil AA, Moeller DS, Nyman J. The HILUS-trial—a prospective Nordic multicenter phase 2 study of ultracentral lung tumors treated with stereotactic body radiotherapy. J Thorac Oncol. 2021;16(7):1200–10.

McDermott RL, Mihai A, Dunne M, Keys M, O'Sullivan S, Thirion P, ElBeltagi N, Armstrong JG. Stereotactic ablative radiation therapy for large (≥5 cm) non-small cell lung carcinoma. Clin Oncol. 2021;33(5):292–9.

Nyman J, Hallqvist A, Lund JÅ, Brustugun OT, Bergman B, Bergström P, Friesland S, Lewensohn R, Holmberg E, Lax I. SPACE–a randomized study of SBRT vs conventional fractionated radiotherapy in medically inoperable stage I NSCLC. Radiother Oncol. 2016;121(1):1–8.

Palma DA, Nguyen TK, Louie AV, Malthaner R, Fortin D, Rodrigues GB, Yaremko B, Laba J, Kwan K, Gaede S, Lee T. Measuring the integration of stereotactic ablative radiotherapy plus surgery for early-stage non-small cell lung cancer: a phase 2 clinical trial. JAMA Oncol. 2019a;5(5):681–8.

Palma DA, Olson R, Harrow S, Gaede S, Louie AV, Haasbeek C, Mulroy L, Lock M, Rodrigues GB, Yaremko BP, Schellenberg D. Stereotactic ablative radiotherapy versus standard of care palliative treatment in patients with oligometastatic cancers (SABR-COMET): a randomized, phase 2, open-label trial. Lancet. 2019b;393(10185):2051–8.

Palma DA, Olson RA, Harrow S, Gaede S, Louie AV, Haasbeek C, Mulroy L, Lock MI, Rodrigues G, Yaremko BP, Schellenberg D. Stereotactic ablative radiotherapy for the comprehensive treatment of oligometastatic cancers: long-term results of the SABR-COMET randomized trial. Int J Radiat Oncol Biol Phys. 2020;108(3):S88–9.

Rulach R, Ball D, Chua KL, Dahele M, De Ruysscher D, Franks K, Gomez D, Guckenberger M, Hanna GG, Louie AV, Moghanaki D. An international expert survey on the indications and practice of radical thoracic reirradiation for non-small cell lung cancer. Adv Radiat Oncol. 2021;6(2):100653.

Sarudis S, Karlsson Hauer A, Nyman J, Bäck A. Systematic evaluation of lung tumor motion using four-dimensional computed tomography. Acta Oncol. 2017;56(4):525–30.

Singh AK, Gomez-Suescun JA, Stephans KL, Bogart JA, Hermann GM, Tian L, Groman A, Videtic GM. One versus three fractions of stereotactic body radiation therapy for peripheral stage I to II non-small cell lung cancer: a randomized, multi-institution, phase 2 trial. Int J Radiat Oncol Biol Phys. 2019;105(4):752–9.

Timmerman R, McGarry R, Yiannoutsos C, Papiez L, et al. Excessive toxicity when treating central tumors in a phase II study of stereotactic body radiation therapy for medically inoperable early-stage lung cancer. J Clin Oncol. 2006;24(30):4833–9.

Timmerman RD, Paulus R, Pass HI, Gore EM, Edelman MJ, Galvin J, Straube WL, Nedzi LA, McGarry RC, Robinson CG, Schiff PB. Stereotactic body radiation therapy for operable early-stage lung cancer: findings from the NRG oncology RTOG 0618 trial. JAMA oncology. 2018;4(9):1263-6.

Trovo M, Linda A, El Naga I, Javidan-Nejad C, Bradley J. Early and late lung radiographic injury following stereotactic body radiation therapy (SBRT). Lung Cancer. 2010;69(1):77–85.

Verma V, Simone CB II, Allen PK, Gajjar SR, Shah C, Zhen W, Harkenrider MM, Hallemeier CL, Jabbour SK, Matthiesen CL, Braunstein SE. Multi-institutional experience of stereotactic ablative radiation therapy for stage I small cell lung cancer. Int J Radiat Oncol Biol Phys. 2017;97(2):362–71.

Viani GA, Arruda CV, De Fendi LI. Effectiveness and safety of Reirradiation with stereotactic ablative radiotherapy of lung cancer after a first course of thoracic radiation: a meta-analysis. Am J Clin Oncol. 2020;43(8):575–81.

Videtic GM, Paulus R, Singh AK, Chang JY, Parker W, Olivier KR, Timmerman RD, Komaki RR, Urbanic JJ, Stephans KL, Yom SS. Long-term follow-up on NRG oncology RTOG 0915 (NCCTG N0927): a randomized phase 2 study comparing 2 stereotactic body radiation therapy schedules for medically inoperable patients with stage I peripheral non-small cell lung cancer. Int J Radiat Oncol Biol Phys. 2019;103(5):1077–84.

Yang ZY, Chang Y, Liu HY, Liu G, Li Q. Target margin design for real-time lung tumor tracking stereotactic body radiation therapy using CyberKnife Xsight lung tracking system. Sci Rep. 2017;7(1):10826.

Chapter 7
Digestive System

Ting Martin Ma and Mekhail Anwar

Introduction

Less than 20% of patients with pancreatic cancer present with up-front resectable disease (Boyle et al. 2015; Shaib et al. 2016a), and local failure rate is high with locally destructive disease as the direct cause of death in up to 20–30% of patients (Hishinuma et al. 2006). Higher doses of radiation therapy (RT) have shown more durable local tumor control and even overall survival (OS) (Petrelli et al. 2017; Krishnan et al. 2016; Reyngold et al. 2021). With recent advances in more effective systemic agents (e.g., mFOLFIRINOX) resulting in improved distant metastasis control, local control (LC) becomes increasingly important. Thanks to technical advances in respiratory motion assessment, and treatment planning

T. M. Ma
Department of Radiation Oncology, University of California Los Angeles, Los Angeles, CA, USA
e-mail: tma@mednet.ucla.edu

M. Anwar (✉)
Department of Radiation Oncology, University of California San Francisco, San Francisco, CA, USA
e-mail: Mekhail.Anwar@ucsf.edu

© The Author(s), under exclusive license to Springer Nature Switzerland AG 2023
R. A. Sethi et al. (eds.), *Handbook of Evidence-Based Stereotactic Radiosurgery and Stereotactic Body Radiotherapy*, https://doi.org/10.1007/978-3-031-33156-5_7

and delivery, SBRT has emerged as an effective local therapy with acceptable rates of toxicity. In select cases, it can render initially unresectable disease resectable. Resection rates vary depending on the chemotherapy regimen and SBRT dose/fractionation, but are generally reported to be ~50–65% for borderline resectable pancreatic disease (BRPC) and ~10–25% for locally advanced pancreatic carcinoma (LAPC) (Petrelli et al. 2015; Rashid et al. 2016; Moningi et al. 2015; Mellon et al. 2015). Importantly, patients who eventually underwent resections also have longer median OS (Petrelli et al. 2017; Moningi et al. 2015; Mellon et al. 2015). Compared to conventionally fractionated RT, SBRT has many advantages including biological dose escalation, shorter total treatment time, superior LC, reduced rate of subsequent margin positive resection, and improved quality of life. SBRT further reduces the total number of treatments from 15 fractions with hypofractionated RT to only 3–5 fractions, which makes it more convenient for patients, offers minimal interruption of full-dose chemotherapy, and allows patients to travel to specialized centers to receive care. SBRT bolsters a high LC rate of ~73% at 1 year for inoperable disease in a pooled analysis of 19 trials (Petrelli et al. 2017), and a satisfactory safety profile with acute/late grade ≥3 GI toxicity generally <10% (Petrelli et al. 2017). Dose escalation and MRI-guided adaptive radiation therapy are actively being explored. The role of SBRT is expanding in all subtypes of localized pancreatic cancer, especially in the setting of BRPC and LAPC.

For primary liver cancers (e.g., hepatocellular carcinoma [HCC] and intrahepatic cholangiocarcinoma [ICC]), the preferred treatment modality is surgery with either resection or orthotopic liver transplantation (OLT) (in case of HCC). However, only 20% of HCC patients and 30% of ICC patients are suitable for surgical management at the time of diagnosis (Tse et al. 2008). For the rest of the patients, liver-directed therapies are considered, which are also routinely used for patients with liver metastasis. Historically, liver radiation was mainly limited to the palliative setting, given concern for radiation-induced liver disease (RILD), limited technology to deliver ablative doses, as well as availability of other local therapies such as radiofrequency ablation (RFA) and transarterial chemoembolization (TACE). In more recent years, thanks to the advancement in image guidance technologies, respiratory motion management, and sophisticated planning techniques, more focused high-dose RT can now be safely delivered to primary liver malignancies or metastasis to the liver with SBRT, which is becoming an increasingly utilized tool in the armamentarium in primary liver cancer patients ineligible for surgical resection or transplantation, and in patients with metastasis to the liver. Additionally, in patients with HCC, SBRT can also be used as a tool for bridging to liver transplantation as up to 30% of patients may be removed from the transplant list due to disease progression (Llovct et al. 1999). In the setting of liver metastasis, maintenance of LC and/or ablation with SBRT nearly significantly translates to improved survival (Kang et al. 2010). MRI-guided SBRT and combination with immunotherapy are rapidly evolving frontiers.

Pearls

Pancreatic SBRT

- SBRT, compared to longer course of chemoradiation, is ideally suitable for smaller tumors (generally ≤6 cm) and located ≥1 cm away from bowel (should not be a contraindication if not met) without frank invasion and without grossly positive nodal disease (Palta et al. 2019).
- Tumor invading the duodenum is an absolute contraindication for SBRT due to the risk of potentially fatal gastrointestinal bleeding.
- Stomach and bowel, particularly the duodenum, are usually the dose-limiting normal structures.
- In BRPC or LAPC after chemotherapy, SBRT may be offered to patients with no evidence of metastases,

adequate performance status (ECOG ≤2), and comorbidity profile (including hepatic and renal function).

- In selected patients with metastatic pancreatic cancer, SBRT can be offered for consolidation and/or to allow time off chemotherapy (Lischalk et al. 2018) as locally destructive disease incurs high morbidity and mortality (Hishinuma et al. 2006).

- In selected patients with isolated local recurrence/progression following conventionally fractionated chemoradiation or SBRT, salvage SBRT re-irradiation may be a safe and reasonable option. Those with a progression-free interval of greater than 9 months prior to isolated local recurrence/progression are most suitable.

Liver SBRT

- In recent years, liver SBRT has emerged as an effective and safe modality for treating primary liver cancers not amenable for resection/transplant, bridging to transplant and treating liver metastasis.

- SBRT compares favorably with other local treatment options such as ablation and TACE in terms of LC and OS. SBRT can be combined with other local treatment modalities.

- For HCC, prospective trial data demonstrate that SBRT LC rates at 1 year ranged from 65% to 100%. OS at 1 year ranged from 48% to 78%. Grade ≥3 toxicity ranged from 0 to 38% (Venkat et al. 2017; Murray and Dawson 2017).

- For ICC, a systemic review reported that SBRT LC rate at 1 year was 83% (95% confidence interval [CI]: 77–89%). OS at 1 year was 58% (95% CI: 50–66%) (Frakulli et al. 2019). Biologically effective dose (BED) greater than 80.5 Gy was associated with improved LC and OS (Tao et al. 2016). Toxicities were acceptable and manageable (Frakulli et al. 2019; Tao et al. 2016).

- For liver metastasis treated by SBRT, LC rates at 1–2 years ranged from 67 to 100%. OS at 1 year ranged from 62 to 85%. Grade ≥3 toxicity ranged from 0 to 20% (Mahadevan et al. 2018).
- As a parallel-functioning organ, liver can receive relatively high doses of radiation as long as a sufficient volume of healthy liver tissue is spared.
- Risk of RILD is very low with liver SBRT respecting normal tissue constraints, although liver toxicity is generally higher in patients with HCC compared with liver metastases given the higher likelihood of cirrhosis and poor hepatic function prior to SBRT.
- There is a dose-response relationship in terms of LC for primary liver malignancies and liver metastasis (Tao et al. 2016; Jang et al. 2013; Scorsetti et al. 2015). Therefore, PTV prescription dose should be as high as possible pending dosimetric evaluation.
- SBRT compares favorably with other local treatment options such as ablation and TACE in terms of LC and OS.
- Prognostic factors for better LC after liver SBRT for liver metastases include smaller tumor size, higher treatment dose, and certain histologies (non-GI, melanoma, or renal cell carcinoma) (Mahadevan et al. 2018; Rusthoven et al. 2009; Lee et al. 2009). OS is associated with smaller tumor volume, absence of extrahepatic disease, performance status of 0 or 1, and LC of treated liver lesions (Kang et al. 2010, 2012; McPartlin et al. 2017; Chang et al. 2011).

Workup

Pancreatic Cancer

- **H&P**: Alcohol use, tobacco use, obesity, BRCA, Peutz-Jeghers syndrome, familial atypical multiple mole melanoma syndrome, ataxia telangiectasia.

- **ROS**: Weight loss, epigastric pain, jaundice.
- **Laboratories**: General: CBC, CMP (including LFTs), LDH, and coagulation panel. Pancreas specific: serum CA 19-9, CEA, amylase, lipase.
- **Imaging**: CT abdomen with contrast (pancreatic protocol with arterial and venous phases) or MRI abdomen, ERCP/MRCP/EUS. PET/CT controversial.
- **Pathology**: Biopsy via EUS (preferred), ERCP, or CT guided. Consider stent placement via ERCP for patients with symptomatic obstructive jaundice. MRCP is useful when looking for occult primary.

Hepatocellular Carcinoma (HCC)

- **H&P**: Prior liver disease (e.g., hepatitis B, hepatitis C, hereditary hemochromatosis), alcohol use, aflatoxin exposure, betel nut chewing, nonalcoholic fatty liver disease. Physical exam focused on ascites, encephalopathy, jaundice, bleeding, and cutaneous manifestations.
- **ROS**: Weight loss, early satiety, fatigue, epigastric pain, jaundice.
- **Laboratories**: CBC, CMP (including LFT), LDH, coagulation panel. HBV and HCV serology, serum AFP. Calculate Child-Turcotte-Pugh (CTP) score/class to estimate liver function—5–6 points: class A; 7–9 points: class B; and 10–15 points: class C.
- **Imaging**: Multiphasic liver CT (non-contrasted, arterial, portal venous, and delayed venous phase) +/− hepatic protocol MRI. On CT, HCC is characterized by intense arterial phase enhancement followed by contrast washout in the delayed venous phase. Complete systemic staging with CT of chest, abdomen, and pelvis. PET/CT not routine.
- **Pathology**: For patients at high risk of developing HCC (e.g., cirrhosis, chronic HBV, recurrent/prior HCC), meeting imaging criteria for HCC is sufficient to warrant treatment without a biopsy (Network 2021).

Intrahepatic Cholangiocarcinoma (ICC)

- **H&P**: Physical exam focused on palpable gallbladder (Courvoisier sign) and hepatomegaly.
- **ROS**: Jaundice, pain stools, dark urine, pruritus, weight loss, abdominal pain.
- **Laboratories**: CBC, CMP (including LFT), CEA, AFP, CA 19-9, viral hepatitis serology.
- **Imaging**: Multiphasic abdominal/pelvis CT/MRI with IV contrast. ICC may be difficult to visualize on CT, so MRI may be helpful. Complete systemic staging with CT of chest.
- **Pathology**: Consider biopsy but not always necessary before definitive therapy if clinical and radiographic suspicion is high (Network 2021).

Treatment Indications

Treatment options for common primary upper GI malignancies and liver metastasis are summarized in Table 7.1.

SBRT vs. Other Liver-Directed Locoregional Therapies

- Tumor board discussion in a multidisciplinary setting should be strongly considered when determining the optimal treatment for each individual patient.
- Ideal candidates for liver SBRT: tumor clearly visualized on CT or MRI; CTP class A/B (score ≤8); tumor size ≤6 cm; >700 cm^3 remaining healthy liver volume; >5 mm from bowel, diagram, chest wall, or central liver; <5 liver lesions; limited extrahepatic disease burden; able to tolerate immobilization. Caution should be used for patients with more impaired liver function, e.g., CTP score >8 points, and consider reserving SBRT only as a bridge to transplantation, since increased liver toxicity has been reported in this

TABLE 7.1 Treatment options for pancreatic cancer, hepatocellular carcinoma, intrahepatic cholangiocarcinoma, and liver metastasis

Disease site	Presentation	Recommended treatment
Pancreas	Resectable	Surgery → chemotherapy → RT or chemoRT[a] Chemotherapy ± chemoRT (conventionally fractionated) or SBRT[b] → surgery → chemotherapy → RT or chemoRT[a]
	Borderline resectable and locally advanced (adequate KPS)	Chemotherapy → chemoRT (conventionally fractionated)[c] → surgery[d] Chemotherapy → SBRT[c,e] → surgery[d]
	Locally advanced (poor KPS)/ medically inoperable	Chemotherapy → chemoRT (conventionally fractionated or hypofractionated)[c] Chemotherapy → SBRT[c] SBRT alone[f] Chemotherapy alone
	Metastatic	Palliation with stents, surgical bypass, chemotherapy, RT, and supportive care as indicated; SBRT not indicated except for expedient palliation
HCC	Resectable or transplantable (meets UNOS criteria)	Resection (preferred), transplant (preferred)[g,h]

TABLE 7.1 (continued)

Disease site	Presentation	Recommended treatment
	Unresectable	Transplant (preferred)[h] or locoregional therapies[i] if not transplant candidate
	Liver-confined disease, medically inoperable	Locoregional therapies[i]
	Metastatic disease	Clinical trial, systemic therapy, or best supportive care; locoregional therapies can be considered in oligometastatic settings or for palliation of pain
ICC	Resectable	Consider staging laparoscopy; resection and regional lymphadenectomy
	Unresectable or metastatic disease	Systemic therapy, locoregional therapies[i], clinical trial; locoregional therapies can be considered in oligometastatic settings or for palliation of pain
Liver metastasis		Locoregional therapies[i], systemic therapy, clinical trial

HCC hepatocellular carcinoma; *ICC* intrahepatic cholangiocarcinoma; *SBRT* stereotactic body radiation therapy; *RT* radiation; *chemoRT* chemoradiation; *KPS* Karnofsky performance scale; *UNOS* United Network for Organ Sharing

[a] Consider adjuvant RT for positive margin, positive lymph nodes, or pT3–T4 disease

[b] Consider neoadjuvant therapy for high-risk patients: imaging findings, very high elevated CA 19-9, large primary tumors, large regional lymph nodes, excessive weight loss, extreme pain (Tempero et al. 2021)

(continued)

TABLE 7.1 (continued)

[c] If no evidence of systemic progression. Otherwise, consider palliative radiation therapy

[d] If deemed resectable after neoadjuvant therapy

[e] Controversial and benefit of preoperative SBRT uncertain. See discussion regarding Alliance A021501 trial in the Evidence section

[f] If chemotherapy is contraindicated or high risk of unacceptable toxicity from chemotherapy. Following surgical resection of pancreatic cancer, adjuvant SBRT is only recommended on a clinical trial or registry (Palta et al. 2019; Rwigema et al. 2012)

[g] Patients with Child-Turcotte-Pugh class A liver function, who are surgically resectable and also fit UNOS criteria, could be considered for resection or transplant. There is controversy over preferred initial treatment strategy (Network 2021)

[h] Locoregional therapies can be considered as bridging therapies before transplantation (Sapisochin et al. 2017)

[i] Commonly used locoregional therapies include ablation (microwave or RFA, cryoablation, percutaneous alcohol injection), TACE, yttrium-90 (^{90}Y) radioembolization (RE), EBRT (such as SBRT), and liver brachytherapy

cohort (Murray and Dawson 2017; Lasley et al. 2015; Andolino et al. 2011). Ultimately, meeting dose constraints is the most important factor in determining eligibility and dose/fractionation.

- RFA not appropriate for tumors next to large vessels (heat-sink), near bowel (bowel damage) or diaphragm (difficulty accessing), and >2 cm (worse LC).
- TACE not appropriate in the presence of venous tumor thrombus (ischemia risk); lower LC rate compared to SBRT (see Evidence below) and generally not considered a curative modality.
- Percutaneous ablation generally outperforms TACE, particularly for smaller HCC tumors (Kim et al. 2014; Hsu et al. 2011).

Radiosurgical Technique

Simulation and Field Design

- ■ **Simulation**
  Pancreatic SBRT
  - ■ Fiducial markers placed via EUS guidance prior to CT simulation.
  - ■ At least 2-h NPO. Supine with arms up. Immobilization with a custom cradle ± wing board. Thin-sliced CT scan with IV contrast. Small amount (<3 oz) of oral contrast (e.g., omnipaque) ~20 min before simulation can be considered to better visualize the small bowel.
  - ■ 4D-CT can be used at the time of simulation to quantify respiratory motion. Should the tumor exhibit >3 mm of motion with respiration on 4D-CT, motion management techniques such as monitored breath-hold, active breathing control, tumor tracking/gating, or compression belt should be considered (Narang 2018). End exhalation position may be more reproducible than inhalation positions. Two sequential breath-hold scans can be used to assess the repeatability of motion management and construction of an individualized PTV.
  - ■ For patients simulated without breath-hold, 4D-CT simulation is recommended.
  - ■ MRI simulation to improve visualization when utilizing MRI-guided radiation therapy (MRgRT).

  Liver SBRT
  - ■ Consider fiducial marker placement prior to simulation if location cannot be accurately ascertained on daily imaging. Surgical clips, calcifications, or lipiodol from prior TACE procedures can also be used as surrogate markers if appropriate and fixed in place. Stents and catheters should be used with greater caution as they may migrate.

- Supine, arms above head, Vac-Lok, or alpha cradle to stabilize torso.
- HCC: Multiphasic IV contrast recommended for the planning CT. ICC and liver metastasis: arterial phase CT scan not typically needed. If using MR-guided RT (MRgRT), perform MRI simulation with IV Eovist contrast and fiducial markers are not needed.
- Breath-hold (exhale breath-hold preferred for greater reproducibility; however, inhale is acceptable if exhale cannot be performed), active breathing control, or abdominal compression preferred to minimize respiratory motion. A 4D-CT scan is needed to measure liver motion when respiratory management is not feasible (McPartlin et al. 2017).
- Oral contrast may aid in delineating stomach and duodenum.
- H2 antagonists or proton pump inhibitors should be given prophylactically to mitigate gastric toxicity.

- **Target delineation**
  Pancreatic SBRT
  - GTV should be delineated based on simulation CT, diagnostic dual-phase CT, PET/CT, and diagnostic MRI abdomen (if available, or simulation MRI if MRgRT is planned).
  - MRI-based contouring recommendations for GTV and OARs have been published by Heerkens et al. (2017).
  - Considerable variability exists among institutions regarding target delineation. Generally, if breath-hold (or other motion management strategy) is used, iGTV can be created from appropriate phases accounting for variability in tumor position among the breath-hold scans. If 4D-CT is used, an ITV can be created to capture the extent of tumor during all phases of respiration. If both 4D-CT and breath-hold are used, contour GTV based on the phase

from 4D-CT that most closely matches with breath-hold contrast scan (e.g., typically around 50% if matching to an exhale breath-hold scan). Then, contour iGTV/ITV based on maximum intensity projection (MIP) sequence and check against images of each individual respiratory phase to ensure capturing the full extent of tumor. OARs can be contoured based on the mean or an ITV of OARs can be used instead.

■ PTV is typically defined as the GTV/iGTV with a 2–5 mm margin (Moningi et al. 2015; Mellon et al. 2015; Rajagopalan et al. 2013; Koay et al. 2020), although a recent study suggests that this margin may not be enough (Han-Oh et al. 2021). At the UCSF, for 4D-CT or exhale breath-hold scan, to generate PTV, a radial 5 mm expansion and 8 mm superior/inferior margin of iGTV/ITV are used. For inhale breath-hold scan, given increased instability, a larger PTV (e.g., 8 mm radial and 1 cm superior/inferior) can be considered. When necessary, a modified PTV (mPTV) can be generated by sub-tracting the critical structures such as bowel. Alternatively, PTV contour is not modified in the planning process; rather one accepts that the over-lapping region of the PTV with OAR/planning organ at risk volume (PRV) will be underdosed while still covering the rest of the PTV to the maxi-mal extent possible. Consider delineating tumor-vessel interface (TVI), particularly the superior mesenteric vein (SMV), as regions of simultaneous integrated boost (SIB). Approximately one-third of patients who had locoregional recurrences after SBRT recurred near the celiac trunk and superior mesenteric artery (SMA) (Koay et al. 2020).

■ PRV is typically a 2–5 mm expansion on the OARs such as the stomach and small bowel to aid in plan-ning to limit acute and late toxicities. This can be contoured on the average images on a 4D-CT scan.

- If surgical resection is a possibility after SBRT, attention to ensure areas of future anastomosis is spared of high-dose radiation.
- Elective lymph node chains and positive lymph nodes are not typically included in the SBRT field unless the positive nodes are close to the primary tumor. In case of regional lymphadenopathy that is unresponsive to chemotherapy and farther away from the primary tumor, these nodes should be included in the radiation field although a more fractionated approach should be considered.

Liver SBRT

- Liver metastasis: GTV is best seen in the portal venous CT phase and appears hypodense in relation to the liver parenchyma.
- HCC: GTV is delineated based on arterial phase and/or delayed-phase imaging; venous phase helpful for portal vein thrombosis delineation. CT should be registered to a multiphasic liver MRI scan with gadolinium if available.
- HCC: No expansion from GTV to CTV for the majority of cases. Per RTOG 1112, CTV can be expanded to include regions at high risk for microscopic disease (e.g., non-tumor vascular thrombi, prior TACE sites, or adjacent ablation sites).
- No need for ITV if end exhalation or breath-hold techniques are used. But if free breathing is used (not preferred), an ITV can be contoured based on MIP, 4D, or average images.
- PTV = 3-5 mm + GTV (based on individual tumor motion, breath-hold reproducibility, presence of fiducial markers, onboard imaging techniques, etc.). Up to 1 cm if free breathing.
- Consensus contouring guideline for HCC available from RTOG (Hong et al. 2014).

Dose Prescription

Pancreatic Cancer

- BRPC: 30–33 Gy in 5 fractions to the tumor with a consideration for a SIB of up to 40 Gy to the tumor vessel interface (Palta et al. 2019).
- LAPC: 33–40 Gy in 5 fractions to the tumor (Palta et al. 2019).
- At least 95% of the mPTV (excluding luminal OARs) should be covered by the prescription dose with 95% of non-modified PTV receiving 30–33 Gy in 5 fractions. In areas of overlap or proximity to the OARs, lower dose to PTV (c.g., 30 Gy in 5 fractions) might be advisable to meet dose constraints.
- Dose escalation (BED_{10} > 70 Gy) can be considered in selected patients with BRPC or LAPC without distant metastasis; adequate performance status (ECOG ≤2); favorable anatomy in relation to OARs; adequate hematologic, renal, and hepatic function; and reproducible motion management (tumor motion ≤5 mm). Contraindications include prior overlapping abdominal radiation treatment, prior surgical resection of pancreatic cancer, active or uncontrolled gastric or duodenal ulcer, duodenal invasion, therapeutic anticoagulation, and residual or persistent grade 3 chemotherapy toxicity (Koay et al. 2020).
- In dose-escalated SBRT, Koay et al. (2020) defined PTV_low = 3 mm expansion of (iGTV + TVI), PTV_high = PTV_low − PRV. PRV = 5 mm expansion of all bowel structures, including the small and large intestine. Dose to PTV_low was 33 Gy in 5 fractions and dose to PTV_high was 50 Gy in 5 fractions. Aim for TVI to receive 40–50 Gy if dosimetrically feasible.
- Multi-fraction SBRT compared to single-fraction SBRT has significantly lower rates of grade ≥2 GI toxicity without compromising LC or OS (Pollom et al. 2014).

HCC

- Given evidence of likely dose-response relationship in terms of LC and even OS (Jang et al. 2013; Scorsetti et al. 2015), primary HCC should be treated to the highest dose allowed by dosimetric constraints. Scorsetti et al. suggested improved clinical outcomes with BED >100 Gy (Scorsetti et al. 2015). Prescription dose should be based on the volume of liver being irradiated and the risk for RILD/hepatotoxicity. RTOG 1112 recommends dose escalation based on mean liver dose (MLD) as shown in Table 7.2.
- For CTP class A patients: If smaller peripheral tumor, consider 45–54 Gy in 3 fractions pending dosimetric evaluation. If larger lesion or near bowel or central liver, consider 30–50 Gy.

TABLE 7.2 Liver SBRT prescription dose escalation per RTOG 1112

Priority constraint	Prescription dose	
Allowed mean liver dose [MLD] (Gy)	Planned prescription dose (Gy)	If the maximum allowed MLD is exceeded at this planned dose
13.0	50	Reduce to 45 Gy and re-evaluate
15.0	45	Reduce to 40 Gy and re-evaluate
15.0	40	Reduce to 35 Gy and re-evaluate
15.5	35	Reduce to 30 Gy and re-evaluate
16.0	30	Reduce to 27.5 Gy and re-evaluate
17.0	27.5	Ineligible for SBRT

Adapted from RTOG 1112 protocol. MLD, mean liver dose; SBRT, stereotactic body radiation therapy

- For CTP class B patients: Consider 25–40 Gy in 5 fractions.
- Per RTOG 1112, vascular tumor thrombosis (VTT, e.g., portal vein thrombosis) dose should be the same as the primary HCC prescription dose. Lower doses are acceptable if required to maintain normal tissue limits. Non-tumor bland thrombosis is not recommended to be irradiated but may be included as CTV if judged at risk of containing HCC.

ICC

- Tao et al. showed that ablative dose of RT (BED ≥80.5 Gy) is associated with improved LC and OS in inoperable ICC, with long-term survival rates that compared favorably with resection (Tao et al. 2016).
- In their study, radiation dose was the single most important prognostic factor. The 3-year OS rate for patients receiving BED ≥80.5 Gy was 73%; 3-year LC rate was 78%. Higher BED was associated with higher LC and even OS.

Liver Metastasis

- There is strong evidence of improved LC of liver metastases with SBRT dose escalation, so the highest dose allowed by dosimetric constraints should be considered.
- BED ≥75 Gy is associated with improved LC (71% vs. 31%) (Chang et al. 2011). Modeling suggests that BED of 117 Gy would be needed for a 90% LC rate at 1 year (Chang et al. 2011).
- Some series demonstrate that breast cancer metastases are more responsive to SBRT (Klement et al. 2017) while GI histology, melanoma, and renal cell carcinoma are more radioresistant and require higher dose for LC (Chang et al. 2011; Katsoulakis et al. 2014; Stinauer et al. 2011).

- Small peripheral tumors or more radioresistant histologies (colorectal, melanoma, renal cell carcinoma): 45–54 Gy in 3 fractions or as high as dosimetrically feasible (Chang et al. 2011; Katsoulakis et al. 2014; Stinauer et al. 2011).
- Larger tumor, located in central liver or close to OARs: 40–50 Gy in 5 fractions.

Treatment Delivery

Pancreatic SBRT

- Daily image guidance with fiducial markers and volumetric imaging (e.g., CBCT) is recommended.
- Use fiducial markers for pancreas target positioning. Bony anatomy and surgical stents are poor surrogates. If used, larger PTV margins are necessary.
- Adaptive MRgRT can escalate dose to tumors while minimizing dose to normal tissue. Patients receives a volumetric MRI prior to each fraction for daily alignment, and radiation plan is evaluated on the patient's current anatomy. If OAR constraints are not met or if target is under-covered, a new plan can be generated using the same beam angles (adaptive RT).
- Consider using cine imaging (real-time onboard MRI or fluoroscopic imaging) if possible in addition to 2D or 3D image guidance to verify reliable target coverage and for gating.
- Common dose constraints for pancreatic SBRT are shown in Table 7.3.

Liver SBRT

- Gantry-based vs. robotic-based (i.e., CyberKnife) linear accelerator platforms vs. MRgRT. Respiratory management techniques such as respiratory gating,

TABLE 7.3 Dose constraints for pancreatic SBRT

Structure	Fractions	Constraints	Study
Spinal cord	3	Dmax < 18 Gy	Rajagopalan et al. (2013)
	5	V20Gy < 1 cc	Herman et al. (2015)
	6	Dmax < 20 Gy	Comito et al. (2017)
Liver	3	V15Gy < 700 cc	Rajagopalan et al. (2013)
	5	V12Gy < 50%	Herman et al. (2015)
Kidneys	3	V15Gy < 1/3 total volume	Rajagopalan et al. (2013)
	5	V12Gy < 75% (combined)	Herman et al. (2015)
	6	Mean < 10 Gy (each)	Comito et al. (2017)
Duodenum	5	V33Gy < 1 cc	Herman et al. (2015)
	5	V20Gy < 30 cc, V30Gy < 3 cc, V35Gy < 1 cc	Colbert et al. (2018)
	6	Mean < 20 Gy V30Gy < 2 cc, V35Gy < 0.5 cc	Comito et al. (2017)
Stomach	3	Dmax < 30 Gy	Rajagopalan et al. (2013)
	5	V33Gy < 1 cc	Herman et al. (2015)
	5	V20Gy < 20 cc, V30Gy < 2 cc, V35Gy < 1 cc,	Colbert et al. (2018)

(continued)

TABLE 7.3 (continued)

Structure	Fractions	Constraints	Study
	6	Mean < 20 Gy V30Gy < 2 cc, V35Gy < 0.5 cc	Comito et al. (2017)
Small bowel	3	Dmax < 25 Gy	Rajagopalan et al. (2013)
	5	V33Gy < 1 cc	Herman et al. (2015)
	5	V20Gy < 15 cc, V30Gy < 1 cc, V35Gy < 0.1 cc	Colbert et al. (2018)
	6	Mean < 20 Gy V30Gy < 2 cc, V35Gy < 0.5 cc	Comito et al. (2017)

abdominal compression, or breath-hold should be used except for CyberKnife, which is equipped with respiratory tracking during delivery.

- Daily image guidance with orthogonal kV imaging and/or CBCT aligning to soft-tissue surrogate markers for gantry- and robotic-based Linac platforms.
- MRgRT is an emerging effective treatment option given MRI's superior soft-tissue contrast resolution, the ability for real-time image-guided treatment delivery, and online adaptive planning (Feldman et al. 2019; Rosenberg et al. 2019; Boldrini et al. 2021).
- Consider every other day treatment in patients with decreased liver function or when dose to OARs is close to established dose constraints.
- Common dose constraints for liver SBRT are shown in Table 7.4.

TABLE 7.4 Dose constraints for liver SBRT

Structure	Fractions	Constraints	Study
Liver	3	Dmean ≤13 Gy (primary liver disease) or 15 Gy (liver metastasis)	QUANTEC (Pan et al. 2010)
	3	≥700 cm³ of liver to ≤15–17 Gy[a]	(Kavanagh et al. 2006; Schefter et al. 2005)
	3	≥800 cm³ of liver to ≤18 Gy	(Son et al. 2010)
	5	Liver minus all GTVs: >700 cc and V10Gy <70%	RTOG 1112
	5	≥700 cm³ of liver to ≤21 Gy	(Heron et al. 2019)
	6	Dmean ≤ 18 Gy (primary liver disease) or 20 Gy (liver metastasis)	QUANTEC (Pan et al. 2010)
Esophagus	5	D0.5cc < 32 Gy	RTOG 1112
Stomach	5	D0.5cc < 30 Gy	RTOG 1112
	6	D0.5cc < 32 Gy	(McPartlin et al. 2017)
Spinal cord +5 mm	5	D0.5cc < 25 Gy	RTOG 1112
	6	D0.5cc < 27 Gy	(McPartlin et al. 2017)
Kidneys	5	Combined Dmean <10 Gy	RTOG 1112

(continued)

TABLE 7.4 (continued)

Structure	Fractions	Constraints	Study
	6	≤18 Gy to 2/3 of the combined kidneys or 10 Gy to 90% of 1 functioning kidney	(McPartlin et al. 2017)
Duodenum	5	D0.5cc < 30 Gy	RTOG 1112
	6	D0.5cc < 33 Gy	(McPartlin et al. 2017)
Small bowel	5	D0.5cc < 30 Gy	RTOG 1112
	6	D0.5cc < 34 Gy	(McPartlin et al. 2017)
Large bowel	5	D0.5cc < 32 Gy	RTOG 1112
	6	D0.5cc < 36 Gy	(McPartlin et al. 2017)
Central biliary tract[b]	–	$V_{BED10}40 \geq 37$ cc and $V_{BED10}30 \geq 45$ cc	(Toesca et al. 2017)
Heart	5	D30cc < 30 Gy	RTOG 1112
Great vessels	5	D0.5cc < 60 Gy	RTOG 1112
Chest wall	5	D0.5cc < 50 Gy	RTOG 1112
Gallbladder	5	D0.5cc < 55 Gy	RTOG 1112
Common bile duct	5	D0.5cc < 50 Gy	RTOG 1112

Per HyTEC (Miften et al. 2021), mean prescription dose of 50 Gy in 3–6 fractions would result in a grade 3 general GI toxicity risk of <10%

[a] By sparing a volume of 700 cc of normal liver from receiving >15 Gy, no RILD or other severe toxicities were observed (Kavanagh et al. 2006)

[b] Central biliary tract was defined as 1.5 cm isotropic expansions from the portal vein (Toesca et al. 2017)

Toxicities and Management

Pancreatic SBRT

- Acute toxicities:
  - Fatigue, enteritis, gastritis (manifested as nausea/vomiting, anorexia, diarrhea, abdominal pain, dysgeusia), GI bleeding, and elevated liver function tests. Recommend prescribing an antacid or PPI medication as well as antiemetics prophylactically.
  - Rate varies considerably among studies with acute grade ≥3 GI toxicity generally around 0–20%. In a meta-analysis including 19 studies (see below), only 3 studies reported acute grade ≥3 toxicity exceeding 10% (Petrelli et al. 2017).
  - In the study by Herman et al. (see below), in which neoadjuvant gemcitabine → SBRT (33 Gy in 5 fx) gemcitabine for LAPC, acute grade ≥3 toxicity was 12% (2% enteritis, gastritis, ulcer, or fistula and 10% elevated AST/ALT) (Herman et al. 2015).
- Long-term toxicities:
  - Enteritis, gastritis, ulcer, fistula, perforation, and GI bleeding.
  - Can lead to weight loss from malabsorption. Best supportive care.
  - Bowel wall fibrosis leading to adhesions and obstruction, potentially requiring laparoscopy/laparotomy.
  - Pancreatic and adrenal insufficiency potentially requiring exogenous supplementation.
  - Rate varies considerably among studies with late grade ≥3 GI toxicity generally around 0–11% (Petrelli et al. 2017). In many series, grade ≥3 acute/late toxicity rate was 0%.

Liver SBRT

- Acute toxicities: Abdominal pain, fatigue, anorexia, gastritis/esophagitis, diarrhea, nausea/vomiting, elevated liver enzymes, thrombocytopenia, central biliary toxicity (acute biliary edema, obstruction).
- Long-term toxicities: GI bleed, hepatic or biliary toxicity (biliary stricture, secondary infection).
- Radiation-induced liver injury (RILD): First observed in patients who underwent whole-liver RT. Classic RILD involves the triad of anicteric hepatomegaly, ascites, and elevated liver enzymes, especially alkaline phosphatase ($\geq 2\times$ upper limit of normal or baseline value). Can occur in patients with otherwise relatively well-functioning pretreatment livers. Treatment options are limited, and liver failure and death can result. Nonclassic RILD: general decline in liver function (worsening of CTP score by 2 or more), markedly elevated transaminases ($>5\times$ upper limit of normal or CTCAE grade 4 levels in patients with baseline values $>5\times$ upper limit of normal), or jaundice, 1 week and 3 months after therapy. More commonly occur in HCC patients with poor liver function. CTP score is comprised of five variables: albumin, bilirubin, INR, ascites, and encephalopathy.
- Liver metastasis: Grade ≥ 3 toxicity associated with SBRT is generally 1–10%. Most prospective studies reported no or <1% incidence of RILD (Scorsetti et al. 2014).
- HCC patients are more likely to develop radiation-related toxicity, due in part to their underlying disease and comorbidities, but still classic RILD is uncommon. However, 20–30% patients had a decline in CTP class 3 months after SBRT (Andolino et al. 2011; Bujold et al. 2013).
- Concurrent systemic therapies, especially chemotherapy and targeted therapies, should be avoided given

concern for increased toxicity with this combination. Unanticipated toxicities may arise when combining SBRT and angiogenesis-targeting agents (e.g., VEGF inhibitors), particularly of late luminal gastrointestinal toxicities (Pollom et al. 2015).

■ Subsequent Y-90 radioembolization should be cautioned given increased risk for radioembolization-induced liver disease (Lam et al. 2013).

Recommended Follow-Up

■ **Pancreatic cance**r: H&P, laboratories, and abdominal CT (multiphasic vs. pancreatic protocol) every 3 months for 2 years, then every 6 months thereafter, to evaluate for disease recurrence/progression.

■ **HCC**: Initial triphasic contrast-enhanced CT or MRI 3 months post-SBRT. For the first 2 years, repeat imaging every 3–6 months and then every 6–12 months (or liver US every 6 months) thereafter (Bruix and Sherman 2011). Notably, the incidence of arterial hypervascularity of the irradiated non-tumor hepatic parenchyma may gradually increase until 6 months after SBRT (to 54% per Park et al. 2014), which may be confused with tumor progression. SBRT-related changes display lack of washout on the delayed phase in the hypervascular area while residual/recurred HCC does not.

■ **Liver metastasis**: Single venous-phase contrasted CT. PET/CT may be helpful for lesions that are initially FDG avid.

■ **Common to liver SBRT**: AFP every 3 months for the first 2 years, and then every 6–12 months thereafter if initially elevated. Closely follow up liver function after SBRT for HCC as up to 30% of patients with locally advanced HCC can have a decrease in their CTP score after SBRT.

Evidence

Pancreatic SBRT

- ■ **SBRT following chemotherapy for BRPC and LAPC in the neoadjuvant setting**
  - ■ *Johns Hopkins* (Moningi et al. 2015): Retrospective single-institution experience with 88 patients (LAPC [84%] and BRPC) treated from 2010 to 2014 with SBRT following gemcitabine-based (72%) or FOLFIRINOX regimens. SBRT doses ranged from 25 to 33 Gy in 5 fractions. Nineteen patients (79% with LAPC) underwent surgical resection, and 84% had margin-negative resections. 20% of LAPC patients underwent surgical resection. One-year LC rate 61%. Median OS 18.4 months for LAPC patients. Resected patients had a median OS of 20.2 months, compared to 12.3 months for unresected cases. Treatment was well tolerated with an acute grade ≥3 GI toxicity rate of 3.4% with one case of grade 4 GI bleeding. Late grade ≥2 GI toxicity in 5.7% of patients with one grade 5 toxicity.
  - ■ *Johns Hopkins/Stanford* (Herman et al. 2015): Phase II multi-institutional trial of 49 patients with LAPC receiving gemcitabine followed by SBRT (33 Gy in 5 fractions), followed by maintenance gemcitabine until disease progression or toxicity. Acute and late grade ≥2 gastritis, fistula, enteritis, or ulcer toxicities were 2% and 11%, respectively. Global quality-of-life scores not changed from baseline to after SBRT. Median OS was 13.9 months. One- and 2-year OS rates were 59% and 18%. LC at 1 year was 78%. 8% underwent margin-negative and lymph node-negative surgical resections.
  - ■ *Moffitt* (Mellon et al. 2015): Retrospective single-institution experience with 159 patients (69% BRPC and 31% LAPC) underwent neoadjuvant chemotherapy for 2–3 months (regimen at physi-

cian's discretion) followed by SBRT (28–30 Gy [median 30 Gy] to the PTV with SIB up to 50 Gy [median 40 Gy] in 5 consecutive daily fractions). For BRPC patients who completed neoadjuvant therapy, resection and R0 resection rates were 51% and 96%, respectively. For BRPC patients who underwent surgery, 7% had a pCR. Median OS was 19.2 months for BRPC patients and 15.0 months for LAPC patients. Surgically resected patients had significantly longer OS (34.2 vs. 15.0 months). 24% LAPC patients receiving FOLFIRINOX chemotherapy underwent R0 resection. For patients not undergoing resection after SBRT, 1-year LRC was 78%. Any grade ≥3 potentially radiation-related acute/late toxicity rate was 7%.

- *Milan* (Comito et al. 2017): Phase II single-institutional study of 45 patients with unresectable LAPC who underwent SBRT (45 Gy in 6 fractions). 71% patients received chemotherapy before SBRT. LC at 1 year was 87% and at 2 years was 90%. Median PFS and OS were 8 and 13 months, respectively. No acute or late grade ≥3 toxicities.

- *Meta-analysis* (Petrelli et al. 2017): Meta-analysis of SBRT in LAPC including 19 studies published in 2005–2015, encompassing 1009 patients. Six were prospective and 13 were retrospective case series. Chemotherapy was administered before and/or after SBRT in 18/19 studies. All studies utilized 4D-CT scan or motion tracking with majority of the studies using fiducial markers. Pooled 1-year OS was 51.6% and the median OS was 17 months (range 5.7–47 months). LRC at 1 year was 72.3%. Overall, acute grade ≥3 GI toxicity ranged 0–36% with only 3 studies reporting >10%. Late grade ≥3 toxicity ranged 0–11% (0% reported in 6 series). Total SBRT dose and higher number of fractions were associated with increased 1-year LRC.

- *Alliance A021501* (abstract from Katz et al. 2017, 2021): Phase II multi-institutional trial studying neoadjuvant mFOLFIRINOX with or without RT in BRPC. 126 patients randomized to eight cycles of neoadjuvant mFOLFIRINOX (n = 70) or seven cycles of mFOLFIRINOX followed by SBRT (33–40 Gy in 5 fractions with 40 Gy limited to TVI as an SIB) or hypofractionated image-guided RT (HIGRT, 25 Gy in 5 fractions) (n = 56) (Wild et al. 2013). Among 40 patients who received RT, 35 received SBRT and 5 received HIGRT. Patients without disease progression proceeded to surgery and then four cycles of adjuvant mFOLFOX6. Eighteen-month OS rate was 67.9% without RT and 47.3% with RT. Among patients who underwent pancreatectomy, 18-month OS rates were 93.1% and 78.9% without RT and with RT, respectively. 48% of patients without RT underwent pancreatectomy vs. 35% with RT. The rate of R0 pancreatectomy was 42% without RT vs. 25% with RT. The trial suggests that preoperative SBRT in an unselected patient population with neoadjuvant mFOLFIRINOX may not be helpful. One criticism of the trial is inadequate RT dose in patients who received HIGRT.

- **Re-irradiation**
  - *Johns Hopkins/Stanford* (Wild et al. 2013): Retrospective dual-institution experience examining the safety, efficacy, and palliative capacity of re-irradiation with SBRT for 18 patients with isolated local recurrence after prior radiation. Fifteen had resection with neoadjuvant or adjuvant chemoradiation and three received definitive chemoradiation for LAPC. Median chemoradiation dose was 50.4 Gy in 28 fractions. Salvage SBRT with a median dose of 25.0 Gy in 5 fractions. Median survival from SBRT was 8.8 months. Local progression <9 months after surgery/definitive chemoradiation is a negative predictor for OS (3.4 vs. 11.3 months) and PFS (3.2 vs. 10.6 months) after SBRT. LC rates

at 6 and 12 months after SBRT were 78% and 62%, respectively. 57% of patients with abdominal or back pain prior to SBRT achieved effective symptom palliation. 28% experienced grade 2 acute toxicity, but none had grade ≥3 acute toxicity. 6% had grade 3 late toxicity in the form of small bowel obstruction.

- *Pittsburg* (Sutera et al. 2018): Retrospective single-institution experience including 38 patients with local recurrence/progression following prior RT. Prior RT median dose 50.4 Gy in 28 fractions. SBRT was delivered to a median dose of 24.5 Gy in 1–3 fractions. At initial diagnosis, 55% of patients were resectable, 8% BRPC, and 37% LAPC. 52.6% of patients had prior surgery. Median OS from diagnosis was 26.6 months with 2-year OS of 53.0%. Median survival from SBRT was 9.7 months. Two-year local and regional control rates were 58% and 82%, respectively. 18.4% and 10.5% experienced late grade ≥2 and grade ≥3 toxicity, respectively. Univariate analysis showed that inferior 2-year LC was significantly associated with post-SBRT CA19-9.

- **Dose escalation**
  - *Emory* (Shaib et al. 2016b): A single-institution phase I study of SBRT dose escalation including 13 BRPC patients after four cycles of modified FOLFIRINOX. Dose to the PTV was 30 or 36 Gy in 3 fractions with SIB dose to the posterior margin (PM) escalating from 6 to 9 Gy. No dose-limiting toxicities were observed, including treatment-related grade 3 or 4 toxicities. Eight patients proceeded to resection (R0 resection in the PM), and five did not due to disease progression. At a median follow-up of 18 months, four patients were alive, and three of the four were disease free. Median OS for resected patients was not reached. SBRT dose of 36 Gy with a 9 Gy SIB to the PM (total 45 Gy) delivered in 3 fractions was safe and well tolerated.

- *MR-linac consortium* (Koay et al. 2020): Provided a detailed description of practical approaches to dose escalation in pancreatic cancer in 15-fraction hypofractionated RT and 5-fraction SBRT (50 Gy) with details in patient selection, target volumes, organs at risk, dose constraints, and specific considerations regarding quality assurance. Gross tumor plus TVI was treated to 33 Gy in 5 fractions. This volume minus 5 mm expansion of bowel structures was boosted to 50 Gy in 5 fractions.

- *MSKCC* (Reyngold et al. 2021): Prospective cohort of 119 patients with LAPC (83% with T3/T4 and 51% with node-positive disease) treated with hypofractionated ablative RT (BED ≥98 Gy) after induction chemotherapy. Dose/fractionation included 75 Gy in 25 fractions (BED = 97.5 Gy) for tumors <1 cm from stomach or intestines, and 67.5 Gy in 15 fractions (BED = 97.9 Gy) for tumors >1 cm away. Respiratory gating, daily CBCT, and selective adaptive planning (based on weekly review of CBCT) were used. Median OS from diagnosis and RT were 26.8 and 18.4 months, respectively. One- and 2-year OS rates from RT were 74% and 38%, respectively. LC rates at 1 and 2 years were 82.4% and 67.2%, respectively. 8% of patients had grade 3 upper GI bleeding but no higher grade events. The same group has previously shown that RT with BED >70 Gy resulted in superior locoregional recurrence-free survival (10.2 vs. 6.2 months) and OS (36% vs. 19%) at 2 years compared to BED ≤70 Gy RT in a cohort of LAPC patients (Krishnan et al. 2016). Although delivered with hypofractionated RT in this study, the high LC and OS underscore the utility of ablative RT (BED ≥98 Gy), which can be achieved with SBRT with MRI guidance, an emerging technology with early promises (see below).

- **MRI-guided RT**
  - *UCLA* (Rudra et al. 2019): Single-institution experience of 44 patients with inoperable pancreatic cancer treated with MRgRT. Treatment included conventional fractionation (BED_{10} = 56 Gy), hypofractionation (BED_{10} = 83 Gy), and SBRT (30–35 Gy in 5 fractions [BED_{10} = 56 Gy] or 40-52 Gy in 5 fractions [BED_{10} = 78 Gy]). Patients were stratified into high-dose (BED_{10} > 70 Gy) and standard-dose groups (BED_{10} ≤ 70 Gy). PTV = 5 mm isotropic margin from GTV or CTV. High-dose patients had significant improvement in 2-year OS (49% vs 30%) and trended towards improved 2-year LC (77% vs. 57%). Median OS for high-dose group was 20.8 months. No grade ≥3 GI toxicity occurred in the high-dose group.

Liver SBRT

- **HCC**
  - **SBRT for inoperable HCC**
    - *Indiana University* (Cárdenes et al. 2010): Phase I dose escalation trial of liver SBRT for primary HCC. 17 patients (25 lesions) with CTP A/B, ineligible for resection, 1–3 liver lesions, and cumulative tumor diameter ≤6 cm. Dose was escalated to 48 Gy in 3 fractions in CTPA patients without dose-limiting toxicity (DLT). Two patients with CTP B disease developed grade 3 hepatic toxicity at the 42 Gy in 3-fraction level, and protocol was amended to 40 Gy in 5 fractions for subsequent CTP B patients without DLT. Six patients underwent a liver transplant. LC was 100% with a median follow-up of 24 months. 1- and 2-year OS rates were 75% and 60%, respectively.

- *Indiana University* (Andolino et al. 2011): Phase I/II study of 60 patients with liver-confined HCC treated with SBRT: 60% with CTP A and 40% with CTP B. Median dose for CTP A patients was 44 Gy in 3 fractions and 40 Gy in 5 fractions for CTP B patients. Treatment was prescribed to 80% isodose line. Median tumor diameter was 3.2 cm. Two-year LC and OS were 90% and 67%, respectively. Subsequently, 23 patients underwent transplant. Two-year OS for transplanted patients was 96% vs. 47% for those who did not undergo transplant. No grade ≥3 nonhematologic toxicities. 12% of all patients with a CTP score ≤7 experienced an increase of >1 grade in hematologic/hepatic dysfunction. Fifty percent of patients with CTP score ≥8 developed progressive liver failure during or shortly after treatment. Half of these patients were treated with the original 42 Gy in 3-fraction regimen, which the authors concluded as unsafe for CTP B patients and abandoned in this population. Authors suggest limiting SBRT for patients with a CTP score ≥8 to those who are already listed for transplant. For those patients not listed for transplant, SBRT may be safe for those with 1–3 lesions, maximum tumor diameter ≤6 cm, and CTP A or B with score ≤7.
- *Korea* (Kang et al. 2012): Phase II trial with 50 patients with inoperable HCC undergoing SBRT as a local salvage treatment after incomplete TACE. Eighty-two percent were CTP A, 12% were CTP B7, and 10% had portal vein tumor thrombosis. All tumors <10 cm. All patients underwent TACE 1–5 times before SBRT. SBRT dose 42–60 Gy in 3 fractions (median dose 57 Gy). 94% of patients with tumor <5 cm received 51–69 Gy; half of the patients with tumor size >5 cm received 42–48 Gy, and the other half received 51–60 Gy. Thirty-eight per-

cent achieved CR within 6 months of completing of SBRT, and 38% had PR. Two-year LR was 94.6% and OS was 68.7%. Two-year LC was 100% for patients receiving >54 Gy. Larger tumor (>5 cm) and lower dose (≤54 Gy) are associated with worse LC. 6.4% had grade 3 GI toxicity, and 4.3% had grade 4 gastric ulcer perforation.

- *Princess Margaret Hospital* (Bujold et al. 2013): Sequential phase I/II trial of SBRT for HCC unsuitable for standard locoregional therapies. 102 patients, all had CTP A disease with ≥700 cm^3 of non-HCC liver. All but 7% had underlying liver disease (HBV, HCV, alcohol related, etc.), and half had prior therapies. Median tumor volume was 117 mL with VTT in 55% and extrahepatic disease in 12%. SBRT dose 24–54 Gy in 6 fractions. LC and OS at 1 year were 87% and 55%, respectively. Median OS was 17.0 months, and VTT was a significant predictor. SBRT dose correlated with LC at 1 year. Toxicity grade ≥3 in 30% of patients and 7 deaths were probably related to RT. 29% of patients had a deterioration of CTP class 3 months after treatment.

■ **SBRT vs. other modalities in HCC**

- SBRT vs. RFA, *University of Michigan* (Wahl et al. 2016): Compared RFA (*n* = 161) and SBRT (*n* = 63) for small-sized HCC (median 1.8 cm vs. 2.2 cm). One-year freedom from local progression for tumors treated with RFA was 83.6% vs. 97.4% treated with SBRT. Increasing tumor size predicted for decreased freedom from local progression in lesions treated with RFA, but not with SBRT. For tumors >2 cm, there was decreased freedom from local progression for RFA compared with SBRT suggesting that SBRT is more effective for larger tumors. Acute grade ≥3 complications were not statistically different (11% with RFA and 5% with SBRT).

- SBRT vs. TACE, *University of Michigan* (Sapir et al. 2018): Compared TACE (*n* = 84) vs. SBRT (*n* = 125) in patients with 1–2 HCC. SBRT patients were older with smaller tumors (2.3 vs. 2.9 cm) and less frequently underwent transplantation. One- and 2-year LC rates were 97% and 91% with SBRT, and 47% and 23% for TACE. Grade ≥3 toxicity 13% (TACE) vs. 8% (SBRT). No difference in OS between groups.
- SBRT vs. surgery, *China* (Su et al. 2017): Compared SBRT (*n* = 82) vs. resection (*n* = 35) for small HCC ≤5 cm, 1–2 lesions with CTP A. The 1-, 3-, and 5-year OS rates were 96%, 82%, and 70% in the SBRT group and 94%, 83%, and 64% in the resection group, respectively. The 1-, 3-, and 5-year PFS rates were 81%, 50%, and 42% in the SBRT group and 68%, 58%, and 40% in the resection group, respectively. None were statistically significant. Similar conclusion was found after propensity score-matched analysis. There was a similarity of hepatotoxicity between the two groups. SBRT ground had fewer complications, such as hepatic hemorrhage, hepatic pain, and weight loss. Acute nausea was significantly more frequent in SBRT patients.

- **ICC**
  - *Korea* (Kang et al. 2012): Retrospective single-institution series with 58 patients (33 ICC and 25 extrahepatic cholangiocarcinoma) with unresectable primary or recurrent cholangiocarcinoma treated by SBRT. 31 patients were treated with robotic-based system and 27 patients with VMAT. The median prescribed dose was 45 Gy in 3 fractions. The median tumor size was 40 cm^3. The 1-year OS rate was 45%, and median OS was 10 months. LC rates at 1 year and 2 years were 85% and 72%, respectively. In multivariate analysis, ECOG score and tumor volume were significant

predictors of OS. In the recurrent tumor setting, >12 months' interval from surgery to recurrence was a positive predictor of OS. 10% of patients experienced grade ≥3 complications (duodenal/gastric ulcer, cholangitis, gastric perforation, bile duct stenosis).

- **Liver metastasis**
  - *International RSSearch® Registry* (Mahadevan et al. 2018): 427 patients with 568 liver metastases from 25 centers. Colorectal was the most common primary. Seventy-three percent had prior chemotherapy. Median tumor volume was 40 mL. SBRT dose was 45 Gy (12–60 Gy) in a median of 3 fractions. Two-year LC better for $BED_{10} \geq 100$ Gy (77% vs. 60%) and better for tumors <40 cm^3 (52 vs. 39 months). Median OS was greater for patients with colorectal (27 months), breast (21 months), and gynecological (25 months) metastases compared to lung (10 months), other GI (18 months), and pancreatic (6 months) primaries. OS was significantly better with smaller tumors (< 40 cm^3) and $BED_{10} \geq 100$ Gy (27 vs. 15 months). No difference in LC based on histology of the primary tumor.
  - *Princess Margaret Hospital* (McPartlin et al. 2017): Long-term outcomes of a prospective phase I and II studies of SBRT for colorectal liver metastases. Of 60 patients treated, 82% had received previous chemotherapy, 23% had undergone previous focal liver treatment, and 38% had extrahepatic disease. The median number of targets per patient was 1 (range, 1–6), and median total target volume was 118 cm^3. The median minimum dose to the GTV was 37.6 Gy (range, 22.7–62.1 Gy) in 6 fractions over 2 weeks. No acute toxicities of grade ≥3, except one grade 3 nausea. With a median follow-up of 28.1 months, no GI bleed or biliary or liver toxicity was seen. LC rates at 1 and 4 years were 50% and 26%, respectively. Increasing minimum dose to the GTV was

associated with improved LC. Lesions receiving a GTV_{min} dose >45 Gy in 6 fractions (75 Gy BED with α/β = 10 Gy) had LC rates of 65% and 49% at 1 and 4 years, respectively, compared to 44% and 14%, respectively, for the remainder. Median OS was 16 months. Smaller total tumor size, no extrahepatic disease, and LC were associated with prolonged OS.

■ **MRI-guided SBRT**
  ■ *Multi-institutional study* (Rosenberg et al. 2019): 26 patients with primary or metastatic liver lesions treated with MRI-guided liver SBRT (6 HCC, 2 cholangiocarcinoma, and 18 metastases). Median dose was 50 Gy in 5 fractions. Breath-hold was used without external respiratory motion management systems. PTV = GTV+ 2-5 mm isotropic expansion. Respiratory gating was used during delivery. Tumor motion was evaluated with a real-time sagittal cine MRI sequence. The 1-year and 2-year OS rates were 69% and 60%, respectively. With a median follow-up of 21.2 months, overall LC was 80.4% (100% and 75% for HCC and colorectal metastases, respectively). No grade ≥4 GI toxicities. The 1-year and 2-year OS rates were 69% and 60%, respectively.

Selected Ongoing Studies

Pancreatic SBRT

■ Selected ongoing studies of pancreatic SBRT are shown in Table 7.5.

Liver SBRT

■ Selected ongoing studies of liver SBRT are shown in Table 7.6.

TABLE 7.5 Selected ongoing studies of pancreatic SBRT

Title	Study population	Phase	Model/ allocation	Regimen	Institution	NCT #	Primary outcome	Date opened	Status
Phase III FOLFIRINOX (mFFX) +/− SBRT in locally advanced pancreatic cancer	LAPC	III	Randomized	mFOLFIRINOX vs. mFOLFIRINOX + SBRT	Stanford University	NCT01926197	1-Year progression-free survival	8/20/2013	Active, not recruiting
Combination chemotherapy with or without hypofractionated radiation therapy before surgery in treating patients with pancreatic cancer	BRPC	II	Randomized	mFOLFIRINOX + surgery + FOLFOX vs. mFOLFIRINOX + SBRT + surgery + FOLFOX	Alliance for Clinical Trials in Oncology	NCT02839343	Overall survival	7/20/2016	Active, not recruiting
Stereotactic MRI-guided on-table adaptive radiation therapy (SMART) for locally advanced pancreatic cancer	LAPC	II	Single arm	Stereotactic MRI-guided on-table adaptive radiation therapy 50 Gy in 5 fractions	Multi-institutional	NCT03621644	Recruiting	8/8/2018	GI toxicity

Table 7.6 Selected ongoing studies of liver SBRT

Title	Study population	Phase	Model/allocation	Regimen	Institution	NCT #	Primary outcome	Date opened	Status
Pembrolizumab and stereotactic radiotherapy combined in subjects with advanced hepatocellular carcinoma – a phase II study	Advanced HCC with disease progression after sorafenib	II	Single arm	Concurrent SBRT (5 fx) with pembrolizumab followed by maintenance pembrolizumab until disease progression or intolerable toxicity	University of Toronto	NCT03316872	Overall response rate	2/15/2018	Recruiting
RTOG 1112: Randomized Phase III Study of Sorafenib Versus Stereotactic Body Radiation Therapy Followed by Sorafenib in Hepatocellular Carcinoma	Primary or recurrent HCC	III	Randomized	Sorafenib alone vs. liver SBRT (5 fractions) + sorafenib	RTOG	NCT01730937	Overall survival	11/21/2012	Active, not recruiting

Title	Study population	Phase	Model/allocation	Regimen	Institution	NCT #	Primary outcome	Date opened	Status
A phase III randomized trial of protons versus photons for hepatocellular carcinoma	HCC	III	Randomized	Proton therapy (5 or 15 fractions) vs. photon therapy (5 or 15 fractions) over 15–24 days	NRG Oncology	NCT03186898	Overall survival	7/14/2017	Recruiting
Phase II of adaptative magnetic resonance-guided stereotactic body radiotherapy (SBRT) for treatment of primary or secondary progressive liver tumors	Primary or secondary liver tumors	II	Single arm	Adaptive MR-guided SBRT (50 Gy in 5 fractions if lesion near OARs; 60 Gy in 6 fractions if lesion far away from OARs)	Centre Georges-François Leclerc	NCT04242342	Local control at 2 years	1/27/2020	Recruiting

References

Andolino DL, Johnson CS, Maluccio M, Kwo P, Tector AJ, Zook J, et al. Stereotactic body radiotherapy for primary hepatocellular carcinoma. Int J Radiat Oncol Biol Phys. 2011;81(4):e447–53.

Boldrini L, Corradini S, Gani C, Henke L, Hosni A, Romano A, et al. MR-guided radiotherapy for liver malignancies. Front Oncol. 2021;11:616027.

Boyle J, Czito B, Willett C, Palta M. Adjuvant radiation therapy for pancreatic cancer: a review of the old and the new. J Gastrointest Oncol. 2015;6(4):436–44.

Bruix J, Sherman M. Management of hepatocellular carcinoma: an update. Hepatology. 2011;53(3):1020–2.

Bujold A, Massey CA, Kim JJ, Brierley J, Cho C, Wong RK, et al. Sequential phase I and II trials of stereotactic body radiotherapy for locally advanced hepatocellular carcinoma. J Clin Oncol. 2013;31(13):1631–9.

Cárdenes HR, Price TR, Perkins SM, Maluccio M, Kwo P, Breen TE, et al. Phase I feasibility trial of stereotactic body radiation therapy for primary hepatocellular carcinoma. Clin Transl Oncol. 2010;12(3):218–25.

Chang DT, Swaminath A, Kozak M, Weintraub J, Koong AC, Kim J, et al. Stereotactic body radiotherapy for colorectal liver metastases: a pooled analysis. Cancer. 2011;117(17):4060–9.

Colbert LE, Rebueno N, Moningi S, Beddar S, Sawakuchi GO, Herman JM, et al. Dose escalation for locally advanced pancreatic cancer: how high can we go? Adv Radiat Oncol. 2018;3(4):693–700.

Comito T, Cozzi L, Clerici E, Franzese C, Tozzi A, Iftode C, et al. Can stereotactic body radiation therapy be a viable and efficient therapeutic option for Unresectable locally advanced pancreatic adenocarcinoma? Results of a phase 2 study. Technol Cancer Res Treat. 2017;16(3):295–301.

Feldman AM, Modh A, Glide-Hurst C, Chetty IJ, Movsas B. Real-time magnetic resonance-guided liver stereotactic body radiation therapy: an institutional report using a magnetic resonance-Linac system. Cureus. 2019;11(9):e5774.

Frakulli R, Buwenge M, Macchia G, Cammelli S, Deodato F, Cilla S, et al. Stereotactic body radiation therapy in cholangiocarcinoma: a systematic review. Br J Radiol. 2019;92(1097):20180688.

Han-Oh S, Hill C, Kang-Hsin Wang K, Ding K, Wright JL, Alcorn S, et al. Geometric reproducibility of fiducial markers and efficacy of a patient-specific margin design using deep inspiration breath hold for stereotactic body radiation therapy for pancreatic cancer. Adv Radiat Oncol. 2021;6(2):100655.

Heerkens HD, Hall WA, Li XA, Knechtges P, Dalah E, Paulson ES, et al. Recommendations for MRI-based contouring of gross tumor volume and organs at risk for radiation therapy of pancreatic cancer. Pract Radiat Oncol. 2017;7(2):126–36.

Herman JM, Chang DT, Goodman KA, Dholakia AS, Raman SP, Hacker-Prietz A, et al. Phase 2 multi-institutional trial evaluating gemcitabine and stereotactic body radiotherapy for patients with locally advanced unresectable pancreatic adenocarcinoma. Cancer. 2015;121(7):1128–37.

Heron D, Huq MS, Herman JM. Stereotactic radiosurgery and stereotactic body radiation therapy (SBRT). 2019.

Hishinuma S, Ogata Y, Tomikawa M, Ozawa I, Hirabayashi K, Igarashi S. Patterns of recurrence after curative resection of pancreatic cancer, based on autopsy findings. J Gastrointest Surg. 2006;10(4):511–8.

Hong TS, Bosch WR, Krishnan S, Kim TK, Mamon HJ, Shyn P, et al. Interobserver variability in target definition for hepatocellular carcinoma with and without portal vein thrombus: radiation therapy oncology group consensus guidelines. Int J Radiat Oncol Biol Phys. 2014;89(4):804–13.

Hsu CY, Huang YH, Chiou YY, Su CW, Lin HC, Lee RC, et al. Comparison of radiofrequency ablation and transarterial chemoembolization for hepatocellular carcinoma within the Milan criteria: a propensity score analysis. Liver Transpl. 2011;17(5):556–66.

Jang WI, Kim MS, Bae SH, Cho CK, Yoo HJ, Seo YS, et al. High-dose stereotactic body radiotherapy correlates increased local control and overall survival in patients with inoperable hepatocellular carcinoma. Radiat Oncol. 2013;8:250.

Kang JK, Kim MS, Kim JH, Yoo SY, Cho CK, Yang KM, et al. Oligometastases confined one organ from colorectal cancer treated by SBRT. Clin Exp Metastasis. 2010;27(4):273–8.

Kang JK, Kim MS, Cho CK, Yang KM, Yoo HJ, Kim JH, et al. Stereotactic body radiation therapy for inoperable hepatocellular carcinoma as a local salvage treatment after incomplete transarterial chemoembolization. Cancer. 2012;118(21):5424–31.

Katsoulakis E, Riaz N, Cannon DM, Goodman K, Spratt DE, Lovelock M, et al. Image-guided radiation therapy for liver tumors: gastrointestinal histology matters. Am J Clin Oncol. 2014;37(6):561–7.

Katz MHG, Ou FS, Herman JM, Ahmad SA, Wolpin B, Marsh R, et al. Alliance for clinical trials in oncology (ALLIANCE) trial A021501: preoperative extended chemotherapy vs. chemotherapy plus hypofractionated radiation therapy for borderline resectable adenocarcinoma of the head of the pancreas. BMC Cancer. 2017;17(1):505.

Katz MH, Shi Q, Meyers JP, Herman JM, Choung M, Wolpin BM, et al. Alliance A021501: preoperative mFOLFIRINOX or mFOLFIRINOX plus hypofractionated radiation therapy (RT) for borderline resectable (BR) adenocarcinoma of the pancreas. J Clin Oncol. 2021;39:377.

Kavanagh BD, Schefter TE, Cardenes HR, Stieber VW, Raben D, Timmerman RD, et al. Interim analysis of a prospective phase I/II trial of SBRT for liver metastases. Acta Oncol. 2006;45(7):848–55.

Kim JW, Kim JH, Sung KB, Ko HK, Shin JH, Kim PN, et al. Transarterial chemoembolization vs. radiofrequency ablation for the treatment of single hepatocellular carcinoma 2 cm or smaller. Am J Gastroenterol. 2014;109(8):1234–40.

Klement RJ, Guckenberger M, Alheid H, Allgäuer M, Becker G, Blanck O, et al. Stereotactic body radiotherapy for oligometastatic liver disease—influence of pre-treatment chemotherapy and histology on local tumor control. Radiother Oncol. 2017;123(2):227–33.

Koay EJ, Hanania AN, Hall WA, Taniguchi CM, Rebueno N, Myrehaug S, et al. Dose-escalated radiation therapy for pancreatic cancer: a simultaneous integrated boost approach. Pract Radiat Oncol. 2020;10(6):e495–507.

Krishnan S, Chadha AS, Suh Y, Chen HC, Rao A, Das P, et al. Focal radiation therapy dose escalation improves overall survival in locally advanced pancreatic cancer patients receiving induction chemotherapy and consolidative chemoradiation. Int J Radiat Oncol Biol Phys. 2016;94(4):755–65.

Lam MG, Abdelmaksoud MH, Chang DT, Eclov NC, Chung MP, Koong AC, et al. Safety of 90Y radioembolization in patients who have undergone previous external beam radiation therapy. Int J Radiat Oncol Biol Phys. 2013;87(2):323–9.

Lasley FD, Mannina EM, Johnson CS, Perkins SM, Althouse S, Maluccio M, et al. Treatment variables related to liver toxicity in patients with hepatocellular carcinoma, Child-Pugh class a and B enrolled in a phase 1-2 trial of stereotactic body radiation therapy. Pract Radiat Oncol. 2015;5(5):e443–e9.

Lee MT, Kim JJ, Dinniwell R, Brierley J, Lockwood G, Wong R, et al. Phase I study of individualized stereotactic body radiotherapy of liver metastases. J Clin Oncol. 2009;27(10):1585–91.

Lischalk JW, Burke A, Chew J, Elledge C, Gurka M, Marshall J, et al. Five-fraction stereotactic body radiation therapy (SBRT) and chemotherapy for the local management of metastatic pancreatic cancer. J Gastrointest Cancer. 2018;49(2):116–23.

Llovet JM, Fuster J, Bruix J. Intention-to-treat analysis of surgical treatment for early hepatocellular carcinoma: resection versus transplantation. Hepatology. 1999;30(6):1434–40.

Mahadevan A, Blanck O, Lanciano R, Peddada A, Sundararaman S, D'Ambrosio D, et al. Stereotactic body radiotherapy (SBRT) for liver metastasis—clinical outcomes from the international multi-institutional RSSearch® patient registry. Radiat Oncol. 2018;13(1):26.

McPartlin A, Swaminath A, Wang R, Pintilie M, Brierley J, Kim J, et al. Long-term outcomes of phase 1 and 2 studies of SBRT for hepatic colorectal metastases. Int J Radiat Oncol Biol Phys. 2017;99(2):388–95.

Mellon EA, Hoffe SE, Springett GM, Frakes JM, Strom TJ, Hodul PJ, et al. Long-term outcomes of induction chemotherapy and neo-adjuvant stereotactic body radiotherapy for borderline resectable and locally advanced pancreatic adenocarcinoma. Acta Oncol. 2015;54(7):979–85.

Miften M, Vinogradskiy Y, Moiseenko V, Grimm J, Yorke E, Jackson A, et al. Radiation dose-volume effects for liver SBRT. Int J Radiat Oncol Biol Phys. 2021;110(1):196–205.

Moningi S, Dholakia AS, Raman SP, Blackford A, Cameron JL, Le DT, et al. The role of stereotactic body radiation therapy for pancreatic cancer: a single-institution experience. Ann Surg Oncol. 2015;22(7):2352–8.

Murray LJ, Dawson LA. Advances in stereotactic body radiation therapy for hepatocellular carcinoma. Semin Radiat Oncol. 2017;27(3):247–55.

Narang AK. Technical aspects of modern radiation therapy for pancreatic adenocarcinoma: field design, motion management, dosing, and concurrent therapy Ann Pancreat Cancer. 2018;1(8).

Network NCC. Hepatobiliary Cancers (Version 3.2021). 2021. https://www.nccn.org/professionals/physician_gls/pdf/hepatobiliary.pdf.

Palta M, Godfrey D, Goodman KA, Hoffe S, Dawson LA, Dessert D, et al. Radiation therapy for pancreatic cancer: executive summary of an ASTRO clinical practice guideline. Pract Radiat Oncol. 2019;9(5):322–32.

Pan CC, Kavanagh BD, Dawson LA, Li XA, Das SK, Miften M, et al. Radiation-associated liver injury. Int J Radiat Oncol Biol Phys. 2010;76(3 Suppl):S94–100.

Park MJ, Kim SY, Yoon SM, Kim JH, Park SH, Lee SS, et al. Stereotactic body radiotherapy-induced arterial hypervascularity of non-tumorous hepatic parenchyma in patients with hepatocellular carcinoma: potential pitfalls in tumor response evaluation on multiphase computed tomography. PLoS One. 2014;9(2):e90327.

Petrelli F, Coinu A, Borgonovo K, Cabiddu M, Ghilardi M, Lonati V, et al. FOLFIRINOX-based neoadjuvant therapy in borderline resectable or unresectable pancreatic cancer: a meta-analytical review of published studies. Pancreas. 2015;44(4):515–21.

Petrelli F, Comito T, Ghidini A, Torri V, Scorsetti M, Barni S. Stereotactic body radiation therapy for locally advanced pancreatic cancer: a systematic review and pooled analysis of 19 trials. Int J Radiat Oncol Biol Phys. 2017;97(2):313–22.

Pollom EL, Alagappan M, von Eyben R, Kunz PL, Fisher GA, Ford JA, et al. Single- versus multifraction stereotactic body radiation therapy for pancreatic adenocarcinoma: outcomes and toxicity. Int J Radiat Oncol Biol Phys. 2014;90(4):918–25.

Pollom EL, Deng L, Pai RK, Brown JM, Giaccia A, Loo BW Jr, et al. Gastrointestinal toxicities with combined antiangiogenic and stereotactic body radiation therapy. Int J Radiat Oncol Biol Phys. 2015;92(3):568–76.

Rajagopalan MS, Heron DE, Wegner RE, Zeh HJ, Bahary N, Krasinskas AM, et al. Pathologic response with neoadjuvant chemotherapy and stereotactic body radiotherapy for borderline resectable and locally-advanced pancreatic cancer. Radiat Oncol. 2013;8:254.

Rashid OM, Pimiento JM, Gamenthaler AW, Nguyen P, Ha TT, Hutchinson T, et al. Outcomes of a clinical pathway for borderline resectable pancreatic cancer. Ann Surg Oncol. 2016;23(4):1371–9.

Reyngold M, O'Reilly EM, Varghese AM, Fiasconaro M, Zinovoy M, Romesser PB, et al. Association of ablative radiation therapy with survival among patients with inoperable pancreatic cancer. JAMA Oncol. 2021;7(5):735–8.

Rosenberg SA, Henke LE, Shaverdian N, Mittauer K, Wojcieszynski AP, Hullett CR, et al. A multi-institutional experience of MR-guided liver stereotactic body radiation therapy. Adv Radiat Oncol. 2019;4(1):142–9.

Rudra S, Jiang N, Rosenberg SA, Olsen JR, Roach MC, Wan L, et al. Using adaptive magnetic resonance image-guided radiation therapy for treatment of inoperable pancreatic cancer. Cancer Med. 2019;8(5):2123–32.

Rusthoven KE, Kavanagh BD, Cardenes H, Stieber VW, Burri SH, Feigenberg SJ, et al. Multi-institutional phase I/II trial of stereotactic body radiation therapy for liver metastases. J Clin Oncol. 2009;27(10):1572–8.

Rwigema JC, Heron DE, Parikh SD, Zeh HJ 3rd, Moser JA, Bahary N, et al. Adjuvant stereotactic body radiotherapy for resected pancreatic adenocarcinoma with close or positive margins. J Gastrointest Cancer. 2012;43(1):70–6.

Sapir E, Tao Y, Schipper MJ, Bazzi L, Novelli PM, Devlin P, et al. Stereotactic body radiation therapy as an alternative to transarterial chemoembolization for hepatocellular carcinoma. Int J Radiat Oncol Biol Phys. 2018;100(1):122–30.

Sapisochin G, Barry A, Doherty M, Fischer S, Goldaracena N, Rosales R, et al. Stereotactic body radiotherapy vs. TACE or RFA as a bridge to transplant in patients with hepatocellular carcinoma. An intention-to-treat analysis. J Hepatol. 2017;67(1):92–9.

Schefter TE, Kavanagh BD, Timmerman RD, Cardenes HR, Baron A, Gaspar LE. A phase I trial of stereotactic body radiation therapy (SBRT) for liver metastases. Int J Radiat Oncol Biol Phys. 2005;62(5):1371–8.

Scorsetti M, Clerici E, Comito T. Stereotactic body radiation therapy for liver metastases. J Gastrointest Oncol. 2014;5(3):190–7.

Scorsetti M, Comito T, Cozzi L, Clerici E, Tozzi A, Franzese C, et al. The challenge of inoperable hepatocellular carcinoma (HCC): results of a single-institutional experience on stereotactic body radiation therapy (SBRT). J Cancer Res Clin Oncol. 2015;141(7):1301–9.

Shaib WL, Ip A, Cardona K, Alese OB, Maithel SK, Kooby D, et al. Contemporary management of borderline resectable and locally advanced unresectable pancreatic cancer. Oncologist. 2016a;21(2):178–87.

Shaib WL, Hawk N, Cassidy RJ, Chen Z, Zhang C, Brutcher E, et al. A phase 1 study of stereotactic body radiation therapy dose escalation for borderline resectable pancreatic cancer after modified FOLFIRINOX (NCT01446458). Int J Radiat Oncol Biol Phys. 2016b;96(2):296–303.

Son SH, Choi BO, Ryu MR, Kang YN, Jang JS, Bae SH, et al. Stereotactic body radiotherapy for patients with unresectable primary hepatocellular carcinoma: dose-volumetric parameters predicting the hepatic complication. Int J Radiat Oncol Biol Phys. 2010;78(4):1073–80.

Stinauer MA, Kavanagh BD, Schefter TE, Gonzalez R, Flaig T, Lewis K, et al. Stereotactic body radiation therapy for melanoma and renal cell carcinoma: impact of single fraction equivalent dose on local control. Radiat Oncol. 2011;6:34.

Su TS, Liang P, Liang J, Lu HZ, Jiang HY, Cheng T, et al. Long-term survival analysis of stereotactic ablative radiotherapy versus liver resection for small hepatocellular carcinoma. Int J Radiat Oncol Biol Phys. 2017;98(3):639–46.

Sutera P, Bernard ME, Wang H, Bahary N, Burton S, Zeh H, et al. Stereotactic body radiation therapy for locally progressive and recurrent pancreatic cancer after prior radiation. Front Oncol. 2018;8:52.

Tao R, Krishnan S, Bhosale PR, Javle MM, Aloia TA, Shroff RT, et al. Ablative radiotherapy doses Lead to a substantial prolongation of survival in patients with inoperable intrahepatic cholangiocarcinoma: a retrospective dose response analysis. J Clin Oncol. 2016;34(3):219–26.

Tempero MA, Malafa MP, Al-Hawary M, Behrman SW, Benson AB, Cardin DB, et al. Pancreatic Adenocarcinoma, Version 2.2021 NCCN Clinical Practice Guidelines in Oncology. J Natl Compr Canc Netw. 2021;19(4):439.

Toesca DA, Osmundson EC, Eyben RV, Shaffer JL, Lu P, Koong AC, et al. Central liver toxicity after SBRT: an expanded analysis and predictive nomogram. Radiother Oncol. 2017;122(1):130–6.

Tse RV, Hawkins M, Lockwood G, Kim JJ, Cummings B, Knox J, et al. Phase I study of individualized stereotactic body radiotherapy for hepatocellular carcinoma and intrahepatic cholangiocarcinoma. J Clin Oncol. 2008;26(4):657–64.

Venkat PS, Hoffe SE, Frakes JM. Stereotactic body radiation therapy for hepatocellular carcinoma and intrahepatic cholangiocarcinoma. Cancer Control. 2017;24(3):1073274817729259.

Wahl DR, Stenmark MH, Tao Y, Pollom EL, Caoili EM, Lawrence TS, et al. Outcomes after stereotactic body radiotherapy or radiofrequency ablation for hepatocellular carcinoma. J Clin Oncol. 2016;34(5):452–9.

Wild AT, Hiniker SM, Chang DT, Tran PT, Khashab MA, Limaye MR, et al. Re-irradiation with stereotactic body radiation therapy as a novel treatment option for isolated local recurrence of pancreatic cancer after multimodality therapy: experience from two institutions. J Gastrointest Oncol. 2013;4(4):343–51.

Chapter 8
Genitourinary Sites

William C. Chen, Alexander R. Gottschalk, and Mack Roach III

SBRT for Clinically Localized Prostate Cancer

Checklist

- **H&P**: Urinary (AUA) symptoms, history of inflammatory bowel or connective tissue disorder, prior RT, prior TURP, comorbidity (e.g., dementia, severe tremor, cardiac comorbidity), pacemaker status, erectile function, bone pain, family history, DRE.
- **Labs**: PSA. For intermediate- to high-risk patients who may receive androgen deprivation (ADT), testosterone, and baseline LFTs.
- **Tissue**: TRUS-guided biopsy with 12 or more cores. MRI-fusion biopsy is ideal especially if suspicious

W. C. Chen (✉) · A. R. Gottschalk · M. Roach III
Department of Radiation Oncology, University of California, San Francisco, San Francisco, CA, USA
e-mail: William.Chen@ucsf.edu; Alexander.gottschalk@ucsf.edu; Mack.Roach@ucsf.edu

© The Author(s), under exclusive license to Springer Nature Switzerland AG 2023
R. A. Sethi et al. (eds.), *Handbook of Evidence-Based Stereotactic Radiosurgery and Stereotactic Body Radiotherapy*, https://doi.org/10.1007/978-3-031-33156-5_8

lesion(s) not sampled. Assessment of percent of + biopsies (% + Bx) and Gleason score (GS) critical. Establish T stage, and assess the presence of large median lobe.

Indications and Workup

- **Low risk**: PSA < 10, GS 6, T1-T2a. Ten-year prostate cancer-specific mortality (PCSM) ~1–2%:
  - Imaging not indicated for workup
  - Favor management via active surveillance, but RP, EBRT, BT, and SBRT are considered appropriate options for selected patients. ADT not indicated.
- **Favorable intermediate risk (IR)**: Any single IR factor (T2b-2c, GS 7, PSA 10–20) and <50% biopsy cores positive (low volume disease). Ten-year PCSM ~5%:
  - Bone imaging not routinely recommended per NCCN guidelines.
  - Pelvic CT or MRI indicated if >10% pelvic nodal risk.
  - Growing evidence for the role of genomic testing for risk stratification but little evidence involving patients treated with SBRT.
  - Treatment is favored; RP, EBRT, BT, and SBRT provide comparable outcomes. Short-term (ST) ADT (4 months) with RT should be considered (especially for favorable IR patients on a case-by-case basis, but excellent outcomes with monotherapy have been reported).
- **Unfavorable IR**: More than one IR factor (T2b–2c, GS 7, PSA 10–20), or GS 4 + 3 disease, or ≥50% of cores positive (high-volume disease). Eight–ten-year PCSM ~5–10%:
  - Bone imaging favored (NM bone scan, NaF PET/CT, or PSMA PET).
  - Pelvic CT or MRI indicated if >10% pelvic nodal risk.

- Treatment indicated; RP, EBRT+ ST ADT, and SBRT provide excellent outcomes. Combination BT + EBRT or SBRT+EBRT are believed to yield higher control rates. ST ADT with RT (4 months) recommended; however, SBRT±ADT well studied.
- **High risk**: PSA > 20, T3–4, GS $\geq$ 8, 8–10-year PCSM ~10–20%. Very high risk = T3b/4 or primary Gleason 5, or 2+ high-risk factors, or >4 cores with GS8+ disease:

  - Bone imaging and pelvic imaging required.
  - Molecular imaging is useful for staging if available (PSMA, fluciclovine/Axumin) and has been studied in a prospective randomized trial:
    - ProPSMA (Hofman et al. 2020): N = 302. High-risk PCa, PSMA PET/CT vs. conventional staging. PSMA was 27% more accurate and changed management 27% of the time versus 5% of the time with conventional staging.
  - Treatment indicated: Favor combination BT + EBRT or SBRT+EBRT with long-term ADT (18–24 months). Prostate-only SBRT is not well studied in this setting and should not be offered off-trial except in extenuating circumstances. For very-high-risk patients, consider referral to medical oncology for discussion of next-generation anti-androgen therapy or chemotherapy (STAMPEDE (Attard et al. 2022), RTOG 0521 (Rosenthal et al. 2019)).

Simulation

- **Fiducial markers**: Recommend TRUS-guided placement of at least three fiducial markers at least 1 week prior to CT simulation (to allow for markers to "settle"). If fiducial tracking with orthogonal X-ray is planned, markers should ideally be at least 2 cm apart (e.g., 2 markers in the base and 1 in the apex).

- **Rectal spacer**: At the UCSF, hydrogel rectal spacer placement is not routinely recommended, as evidence for its clinical benefit is controversial (Hall et al. 2021).
- **Simulation**: Enema on the day of simulation. For robotic SBRT at the UCSF, we simulate with empty bladder due to prolonged treatment time, and full bladder for LINAC SBRT. For combined EBRT+SBRT, simulate with full bladder for EBRT portion. Simulate with alpha cradle or vac-bag for SBRT:
  - At the UCSF, we perform MRI simulation on the same day in the treatment position with a flat patient table.

Contouring, Treatment Planning, and Image Guidance

- **Urethra delineation**: Fusion of MRI/CT images is accomplished by aligning the gold seeds best seen on "3D VIBE T1-weighted gradient echo," or "susceptibility-weighted imaging (SWI)" MRI sequences, to the seeds on CT in order to facilitate accurate delineation of the urethra identified on T2 MRI sequences onto the CT images for treatment planning. If MRI is contraindicated, CT urethrogram at simulation is used to define the urethra.
- **Contouring**:
  - GTV: any lesion visible on MRI, areas of ECE or SVI.
  - CTV: prostate, and proximal 0–20 mm of seminal vesicles, depending on the risk level of the patient for seminal vesicle invasion (SVI). If gross SVI is present, they are incorporated into the target, while carefully sparing nearby bowel, rectum, or bladder.
  - PTV: two common regimens are used at the UCSF based on physician preference:

◻ 38 Gy in 4 fractions (or 19 Gy in 2 fractions as a boost), CTV + 2 mm, 0 mm expansion to spare rectum posteriorly.

◻ 36.25 Gy in 5 fractions to PTV (40 Gy to the prostate volume), CTV + 3–5 mm, reduced posteriorly.

■ Contour should include the penile bulb and urethra (avoidance structures; include portions of the membranous urethra extending into the bulb, and the bladder neck), femurs, rectum, nearby large bowel and small bowel.

■ Double-check MRI-CT fusion and view contours (axial, sagittal, and coronal images) to ensure that they are reasonable, particularly on the simulation CT.

■ **Prescription, schedule, and dose constraints**:

  ■ Monotherapy:

    ◻ 38 Gy in 4 fractions (Jabbari et al. 2012) to PTV, V100% ≥ 95%:

      ■ Rectum Dmax ≤ 100%, V75% < 1 cc; bladder Dmax Dmax ≤ 100%, V75% < 2 cc; urethra 0.1 cc Dmax<120%; prostate V150% < 50% (limit heterogeneity); bowel Dmax ≤ 28 Gy.

    ◻ 36.25 Gy in 5 fractions to PTV, 40 Gy to the prostate volume and areas of GTV (Meier et al. 2018; Zaorsky et al. 2020):

      ■ Rectum V36Gy < 1 cc (up to 2 cc); bladder V40 < 2 cc, V37Gy < 5–10 cc; prostatic urethra V47Gy < 20%; bowel V30Gy < 1 cc; bulb D2% < 28.5 Gy.

  ■ Boost:

    ◻ 19 Gy in 2 fractions (Chen et al. 2021) to PTV, V100% ≥ 95%:

      ■ Dose constraints identical to above 38 Gy/4 fx, and TG 101.

      ■ Pelvic IMRT can precede or follow boost within 2 weeks; typical dose is 45 Gy in 25 fractions. Ideally, a composite plan is created to

ensure no hotspots in OARs. Pay attention to ureters.
- 21 Gy in 3 fractions has been reported elsewhere (Kim et al. 2020).

- **Image guidance**:
  - Cyberknife®:
    - Many published studies have utilized Cyberknife®, with intra-fraction fiducial tracking capability utilizing orthogonal kV X-ray.
  - Gantry-mounted LINAC:
    - LINAC-based SBRT appears to be as safe and efficacious (Dang et al. 2020). Series with intra-fraction reimaging (3× per fraction, Kishan et al. 2019; or up to every 15–30 s with BrainLab® or other real-time tracking system) and without (D'Agostino et al. 2016) have been reported.
- **Treatment considerations**:
  - Consider daily enema, as per RTOG 0938, although our practice has not been to use daily enemas; patients are encouraged to void prior to each RT session.
  - Consider every other day treatment (typical practice at the UCSF), or twice-weekly treatment (based on low-level evidence for possibly lower acute toxicity).
- **Toxicity**:
  - Acute:
    - Genitourinary (mild-moderate: ~30–50%): Urinary frequency and urgency, worsened obstructive symptoms, usually mild to moderate.
      - Management: Tamsulosin or other alpha-blocker, ibuprofen PRN, pyridium OTC PRN for dysuria (obtain UA to rule out UTI), step-up to a short steroid burst (e.g., methylprednisolone dose pack [Medrol Dosepak®]) only if severe symptoms or nearing obstruction. Monitor for urinary obstruction, although rare (<1–3%).

- Gastrointestinal (mild-moderate: ~10–20%): Diarrhea, rarely proctitis, hematochezia.
  - Management: Low-residue diet and anti-diarrheals as needed. ProctoFoam or rectal sucralfate or rectal amifostine can be used for moderate-to-severe proctitis. Hematochezia often a result of aggravated hemorrhoids, but always requires careful history and workup. Biopsy of the rectal mucosa is contraindicated for at least 6 months after radiation and can lead to severe complications.
- Late:
  - Rates of grade 3+ GU/GI toxicity on SBRT monotherapy are <1–3% in a meta-analysis of the literature (Jackson et al. 2019).
    - Rates of grade 3+ GU/GI toxicity are <5%/2% for SBRT boost (Chen et al. 2021).
  - Radiation cystitis, hemorrhagic cystitis, urethral stricture, rectal ulcer, and fistula have been reported:
    - Hyperbaric oxygen can be an effective treatment for late radiation-related toxicities such as cystitis and proctitis. Refer to a certified medical hyperbaric oxygen center staffed with a pulmonologist.
  - Late grade 1 or grade 2 microscopic or macroscopic hematuria is not uncommon (~5–10%), and may require cystoscopy to rule out other causes (e.g., bladder cancer).
  - Erectile dysfunction is similar to conventional and hypofx prostate RT.
  - Factors that may increase late toxicity: prior TURP (ensure accurate avoidance structure contour of the entire TURP defect to avoid hotspots), inflammatory bowel disease, and attempts to cover a large median lobe.

Follow-Up

- Per NCCN v3.2020, PSA every 6–12 months for 5 years, then annually thereafter. DRE annually can be omitted if PSA undetectable.
- Phoenix definition of biochemical recurrence is PSA >2 ng/mL above the PSA nadir:
  - Can consider workup earlier if clear rising PSA on three consecutive tests and based on PSA doubling time.
- PSA bounce (10–20% of patients) can be observed between 6 months and 3 years after SBRT and is usually a "benign" finding.

Evidence

SBRT Monotherapy

- **Pooled meta-analysis** (Jackson et al. 2019): 38 studies with 6116 patients, median f/u of 39 months; 78% of studies included intermediate risk, 38% of studies included a small number of high-risk patients ($N = 470$ pts). Median dose was 7.25 Gy × 5 fractions. Pooled 5-year biochemical control (BC) of 95.3%. Acute/late grade 3+ GU toxicity was 0.5%/2%. Acute/late grade 3+ GI toxicity was 0.06%/1.1%.
- **Pooled multi-institutional data with 7-year results** (Kishan et al. 2019): Ten institutional phase II and two multi-institutional phase II trials were pooled, $N = 2142$ men, 55.3% low risk, 32.3% favorable intermediate risk, 12.4% unfavorable intermediate risk, with median f/u of 6.9 years. Variety of doses (33.5 Gy/5 to 40 Gy/5, 69% Cyberknife). Seven-year biochemical recurrence: 4.5% for low-risk, 8.6% for favorable intermediate-risk, and 14.9% for unfavorable intermediate-risk patients. Seven-year cumulative incidence of grade 3+ GU/GI toxicity was 2.4%/0.4%.

- **HYPO-RT-PC, Phase III RCT, Denmark** (Widmark et al. 2019): N = 1200 patients, tested 78 Gy/39 vs. 42.7 Gy/7 in non-inferiority trial of mostly intermediate-risk (89%) patients. ADT was not allowed. Only ~6% of patients had Gleason 8+, and median PSA was 8.7. SBRT was delivered with a mix of 3D-CRT (80%), IMRT, and VMAT with fiducials. With a median f/u of 5.0 years, SBRT was non-inferior to EBRT (5-year failure-free survival of 84% vs. 84%, HR 1.002, P = 0.99). SBRT had slightly higher acute GU toxicity (28% vs. 23%, grade 2+), but equivalent late toxicity (5% vs. 5%). HRQOL showed higher acute GU/GI symptoms for SBRT, but no difference in late symptoms.
- **PACE-B, Phase III RCT, UK/Canada** (Van As et al. 2019; Tree et al. 2022): N = 874 patients, 91% intermediate risk, no high risk. 36.25 Gy in 5 fractions (40 Gy to prostate) mostly with Cyberknife, versus conventional or moderate hypofractionated RT (most common 78 Gy/39 and 62 Gy/20). No ADT was allowed. Acute RTOG grade 2+ GU toxicity was 23% for SBRT and 27% in the EBRT arms. Acute RTOG grade 2+ GI toxicity was 10% for SBRT and 12% for EBRT. In the study appendix, CTCAE acute GU toxicity appears numerically higher for SBRT (grade 1–2), as were the rates of grade 1–2 diarrhea and proctitis. SBRT symptoms peaked earlier after radiation (2–4 weeks) compared to EBRT (4–6 weeks). Two-year toxicity outcomes showed RTOG grade 2+ GU toxicity in 3% of SBRT and 2% of EBRT patients, and grade 2+ GI toxicity in 3% of SBRT and 2% of EBRT patients. No RTOG grade 4 or higher toxicity was observed at 2 years. Biochemical control and other oncologic endpoints are not yet available but expected to be reported in the next few years.
- **Phase I dose escalation 5-year results, MSKCC** (Zelefsky et al. 2019): N = 136 patients, 32.5 Gy, 35 Gy, 37.5 Gy, and 40 Gy/5 fx. Dose escalation was well toler-

ated. There was a dose-response pattern for greater low-grade toxicity with higher dose. One grade 3 GU toxicity occurred in the 40 Gy arm (stricture). Five-year PSA failure was 15% for 32.5 Gy/5 and 0% for 37.5 Gy and 40 Gy. Rates of 2-year posttreatment biopsy positivity were 47.6%, 19.2%, 16.7%, and 7.7%, for the dose arms. Interestingly, rates of biopsy positivity were higher than PSA failure rates.

- **PSA nadir after SBRT monotherapy versus LDR/ HDR brachytherapy** (Levin-Epstein et al. 2020): $N = 3502$ patients, median f/u of 72 months. 63.5% low risk, 11.7% unfavorable intermediate risk. Nadir PSA was median of 0.2 for SBRT monotherapy at a median of 44 months, between 0.1 and 0.2 for HDR at a median of 37 months, and 0.01–0.2 for LDR at a median of 51 months. There was no difference in biochemical control or rate of PSA <0.4 at 4 years.
- **Key points**: Long-term outcomes are beginning to emerge for SBRT monotherapy for low- to intermediate-risk prostate cancer (Cushman et al. 2019), as well as early results from two phase III studies, HYPO-RT-PC and PACE-B. SBRT can deliver excellent 5–7-year biochemical control rates of 90–95%, with low rates of grade 3+ toxicity of 1–3%. Further study is needed as to optimal treatment for unfavorable intermediate-risk patients, including questions of dose, +/− ADT, and +/− pelvic RT. There is still very limited evidence for SBRT for high-risk patients.

SBRT Boost

- **Georgetown experience** (Paydar et al. 2017; Mercado et al. 2016): $N = 108$ patients with a median f/u of 4.4 years, retrospective review. 54.6% high risk. 19.5 Gy/3 fractions with Cyberknife, plus pelvic IMRT (45–50.4 Gy). Three-year biochemical control was 100%/89.8% for intermediate/high-risk patients.

Toxicity was reported separately; late grade 3+ GU toxicity was 6%, and late grade 3+ GI toxicity was 1% (telangiectasia treated with hyperbaric oxygen). 7% of men had late rectal bleeding.

- **Multi-institutional pooled safety data** (Kaplan et al. 2020): N = 473 patients, retrospective analysis. A variety of doses were used, median 19.5 Gy (fractions not reported). With a median f/u of 33 months, grade 3 GU toxicity was 3.2%, with no grade 4. Grade 3+ GI toxicity was 2.1%.

- **Phase I trial, Asan Medical Center, Republic of Korea** (Kim et al. 2020): N = 26 patients, 100% high risk (mostly very high). Prospective phase I/IIa study. 44 Gy pelvic RT, plus 18 vs. 21 Gy in 3 fractions on Cyberknife. 0% G3+ GU/GI toxicity at a median f/u of 35 months. Three-year biochemical control was 88.1%, with no difference between doses.

- **UCSF experience** (Chen et al. 2021; Anwar et al. 2016): Retrospective analysis of N = 131 men treated with SBRT boost (19 Gy/2, Cyberknife) plus 45 Gy/25 pelvic IMRT, with a median f/u of 73.4 months. N = 101 men treated with HDR boost (19 Gy/2) were used as a comparison. 68.8% of men had high-risk and 26.0% unfavorable intermediate-risk disease; 95% received ADT. Five-year biochemical control (BC) was 88.8% and 91.8% for SBRT and HDR boost. There was no difference in BC or metastasis freedom (5-year 91.7% vs. 95.8%) between SBRT and HDR boost on multivariate analysis or after propensity matching. Grade 3+ GU/GI toxicity was 4.6%/1.5% for SBRT boost. Stricture was not observed in SBRT boost patients and was seen in 1 HDR boost patient. Local failure was 1.7% overall (but low biopsy rate); most recurrences were bone or non-pelvic nodal. Median PSA nadir for SBRT boost was 0.088.

- **Key points**: For unfavorable or high-risk patients, SBRT boost with ADT may offer a safe and effective alternative for those unable/unwilling to receive HDR/

LDR boost. The data is not as robust as for SBRT monotherapy but are accumulating. Data from the brachytherapy boost literature has yet to show a survival advantage to boost therapy but does show a biochemical control advantage over conventional radiation. Comparative trials of SBRT and brachytherapy boost are warranted and ongoing.

SBRT for Prostate Cancer: Oligometastasis-Directed Therapy

Oligometastatic Prostate Cancer

- **Key points:**
  - As the availability of molecular imaging increases, more patients with "oligometastatic" or "oligorecurrent" prostate cancer are likely to be identified. There remains no universally agreed-on definition for "oligometastatic disease." Frequently used definitions limit the number of metastasis to ≤3 or ≤5 extracranial metastases (APCCC 2019 (Gillessen et al. 2020)).
  - For the purposes of accessing prognosis and for management, we find it useful to divide patients into those with "synchronous" (presenting with metastatic disease) vs. "metachronous" (subsequently developed) metastatic disease. Patients with "synchronous oligometastatic" tend to have a worse prognosis, behaving more as the classical metastatic and being at risk for diffuse and/or rapid progression. It is possible that when "oligometastasis" is detected, there is more disease that cannot be detected, i.e., the "tip of the iceberg." In contrast, most of the trials conducted to date (described below) have focused on patients with "metachronous" metastatic disease.

- It is also useful to classify "high-volume" disease metastatic disease as defined in the CHAARTED study: "the presence of visceral metastases or ≥4 bone lesions with ≥1 beyond the vertebral bodies and pelvis …," which has become accepted as a way to describe patients for whom aggressive management (e.g., local treatment) is less likely to be of benefit. Notably, staging in this study was based on conventional, not molecular, imaging. It is important to keep in mind that the number of metastases detected is a function of the sensitivity of imaging modalities used and the volume of disease (and PSA level).
- The appropriate clinical goal of oligometastasis-directed therapy is also yet to be fully defined. Thus far, some studies have focused on non-survival endpoints such as ADT freedom, castrate resistance freedom, and progression freedom. The true rate of "cure" with oligometastasis-directed therapy is unknown but is likely low.
- Further study is needed, and patients should be enrolled on clinical trials of oligometastasis-directed therapy whenever possible.
- Because of the potential of harm with high-dose radiation involved in SBRT, diligent care and clinical judgment must be exercised and an individualized approach to minimize the risk of toxicity depending on body site treated is critical. In particular, SBRT to visceral organs such as lung, abdominal sites close to bowel, and liver can occasionally lead to serious, life-threatening toxicity.

Evidence

- **STOMP, phase II randomized trial** (ASCO 2020 (Ost et al. 2020)): $N = 62$ patients, ≤3 mets by choline-PET, randomized to SBRT/surgery to all sites dz. (met-directed therapy, MDT) vs. observation. SBRT dose was 30 Gy/3 fx; most common surgery was salvage pelvic lymph node dissection (PLND). 54.8% of patients had nodal disease only, and 45.2% had non-nodal (almost all bones). Median f/u 5.3 years, 5-year ADT-free survival 34% in MDT arm vs. 8% in obs. Five-year castrate resistance freedom 76% for MDT vs. 53% for obs.

- **POPSTAR, prospective single-arm trial** (Siva et al. 2018a): N = 33 patients, 1–3 mets by NaF PET/CT + conventional imaging, tx with 20 Gy × 1 (80% isodose) SBRT to all sites of dz. 60.6% bone-only disease. Two-year LC was 93%, and 2-year disease PFS was 39%. Two-year ADT freedom was 48%. 3% ($N = 1$) grade 3 toxicity (vertebral fracture).

- **ORIOLE, phase II randomized trial** (Phillips et al. 2020): N = 54 patients, 1–3 mets (metachronous), no ADT within 6 months and <3 years total, randomized to SBRT MDT vs. observation. PSMA performed but physicians blinded. At 6 months, 19% of SBRT patients progressed (PSA/imaging/ADT initiation) vs. 61% of observed patients. No grade 3+ toxicity. If all PSMA-avid lesions were targeted, progression was lower (16% vs. 63%).

- **Elective nodal RT vs. SBRT for nodal oligorecurrence** (De Bleser et al. 2019): N = 506 patients (309 SBRT, 197 nodal RT [ENRT]), multi-institutional retrospective analysis, with 1–5 nodal oligorecurrence. Median f/u 36 months. Only 8% had prior WPRT, and median PSA at recurrence 2.7. 72% had pelvic nodal oligorecurrence. Pelvic ENRT led to fewer nodal recurrences (20% vs. 42%) due to reduction in pelvic recurrence (1.5% vs. 17.8%). No statistically significant difference in distant nodal, bone, or visceral mets. Three-year castrate resistance freedom was equivalent (88% vs. 87%). Grade 3+ toxicity was 0% for SBRT and 2.5% for ENRT ($P = 0.009$).

- **Safety evidence:**
  - **UK prospective observational trial** (Chalkidou et al. 2021): $N = 1422$ stage IV patients of all primary cancer types (28.6% prostate), 1–3 extracranial metachronous mets (at least 6 months between primary and met development), SBRT 24–60 Gy in 3–8 fx. No treatment-related deaths with median f/u of 13 months. Most common grade 3+ toxicity was fatigue (2%) and elevated liver enzymes (0.6%). One-year OS was 92.3%.
  - **Meta-analysis of prospective trials** (Lehrer et al. 2021): $N = 943$ patients (21 trials) with mixed primary histologies, with ≤5 mets. Acute grade 3+ toxicity was 1.2%, and late grade 3+ toxicity was 1.7%. One-year LC was 94.7%, and 1-year OS was 85.4%. Serious toxicities often involved lung, liver, and bowel.

SBRT for Renal and Adrenal Tumors

SBRT for Renal Cell Carcinoma (RCC)

- **Key points:**
  - Small renal masses (<4 cm) are increasingly identified incidentally on imaging.
  - Traditional signs/symptoms of hematuria, flank pain, and flank mass are typically present for more advanced RCC, and many early-stage RCCs present asymptomatically or with painless hematuria.
  - While the majority of small renal masses are benign, some harbor early-stage RCC:
    - Differential includes RCC, metastasis, lymphoma, abscess, or benign lesions such as oncocytoma, angiomyolipoma, metanephric adenoma, and simple cysts.

- Management of early-stage RCC (T1a–T1b, <4 cm vs. 4–7 cm) should involve a multidisciplinary evaluation including a urologist:
  - Management can include active surveillance, biopsy, partial nephrectomy, or, for inoperable patients, interventional radiology ablation or SBRT.
- There is growing evidence for the efficacy and safety of SBRT for the treatment of early-stage, kidney-confined RCC:
  - Care should be taken for lesions near the renal pelvis and ureter. Comparatively less is known about the safety of SBRT in these areas.
  - Doses most commonly reported include 24–26 Gy in 1 fraction, 40 Gy in 5 fractions, and 42 Gy in 3 fractions. At the UCSF, we favor biopsy for tissue confirmation and fiducial placement for Cyberknife fiducial tracking when feasible.
  - Limiting the high-dose spill (>50% isodose volume) to normal kidney has been suggested to help limit the risk to kidney function.
- Despite having a reputation for being radioresistant, SBRT for both primary and metastatic RCC tumors can achieve good local control and tumor response.

Evidence

- **Meta-analysis of SBRT for RCC** (Correa et al. 2019a): $N = 372$ patients, 26 studies (11 prospective). 26 Gy × 1 or 40 Gy/5 fx was the most common fractionation. Pooled local control was 97.2%, and tumors were generally 2–5 cm, with some studies treating larger, T1b tumors. Tissue confirmation of RCC was obtained in 78.9% of patients. Grade 3–4 toxicity was 1.5%, and change in eGFR was −7.7 mL/min (95% CI −12.5 to −2.8). These toxicities compare favorably to IR ablation. 2.9% of patients (with preexisting renal failure) went on to require dialysis.

- **SBRT for RCC in solitary kidney** (Correa et al. 2019b): N = 81 patients with solitary kidney, underwent SBRT for RCC (histologically confirmed in 91%), median tumor size was 3.7 cm, and 37% were larger than 4 cm. Median dose was 25 Gy/1 fraction. With median 2.57 years' f/u, 2-year LC was 97%, PFS was 77.5%, and cancer-specific survival was 98.2%. Median eGFR decline after SBRT was only -5.8 ± 10.8 mL/min. No patients went on to require dialysis.

- **Pooled multi-institutional retrospective analysis** (Siva et al. 2018b): N = 223 patients, median f/u 2.6 years, mean tumor size 4.4 cm, most patients got 25 Gy × 1 or 40 Gy/5 fx. Grade 3–4 toxicity rate was 1.4%. Two-year local control was 97.8%, cancer-specific survival was 95.7%, and PFS was 77.4%. Mean decrease in eGFR was -5.5 ± 13.3 mL/min.

- **SBRT for T1b (>4 cm) RCC** (Siva et al. 2020): N = 95 patients, median f/u 2.7 years, 78% inoperable. 0% grade 3–5 toxicity. Median dose was 26 Gy in 1 fraction, but ~49% received multi-fraction. Two-year local failure was 2.9%, 2-year CSS was 96.1%, and PFS was 81.0%. eGFR change was -7.9 ± 11.3 mL/min. 20% actually had an increase in eGFR. 17.8% without baseline CKD went on to meet CKD criteria during follow-up, but it was unclear what contribution SBRT had to this. Mean pre-SBRT eGFR was 57.2 mL/min, consistent with grade 3 CKD. 3.2% of patients went on to require dialysis, a rate similar to those reported for partial nephrectomy and IR ablation; attribution to underlying CKD progression versus treatment effect is unclear.

- **SBRT dose and renal function decline** (Siva et al. 2016): N = 21 patients, GFR measured before and after SBRT with Cr-EDTA or Tc-99-DMSA SPECT. Greater GFR decline was reported for 26 Gy × 1 than 42 Gy/3 fx. The R50% conformality index seemed to also correlate with GFR decline. The authors suggest sparing functional kidney from high dose (>50% isodose) to limit GFR decline.

- **SABR-ORCA, meta-analysis of SBRT for metastatic RCC** (Zaorsky et al. 2019): $N = 1602$ patients in 28 studies of SBRT for both extracranial and intracranial RCC metastases. Median treatment volume was 59.7 cc for extracranial mets and 2.3 cc for intracranial. One-year LC was 89% and 90% for extra/intracranial mets. One-year OS was 86.8% for patients with extracranial mets and 49.7% for those with intracranial mets. Grade 3+ toxicity was 0.7% for extracranial and 1.1% for intracranial disease. Authors conclude that SBRT was highly efficacious and safe for metastasis-directed therapy in RCC. Single-fraction tx and higher dose were associated with LC.

SBRT for Adrenal Gland Metastases

- **Key points:**
  - The adrenal glands are common sites for metastasis from non-small cell lung cancer, melanoma, renal cell carcinoma, and colon cancer.
  - When carefully performed, SBRT can achieve good rates of local control with low risk of toxicity. Care must be taken and an individualized approach to each patient's anatomy and nearby organs at risk, in particular bowel, stomach, liver, and kidney:
    - At the UCSF, 50 Gy in 5 fractions (BED-10 of 100 Gy) is a common fractionation, but the dose fractionation is individualized based on target size and nearby structures. Fiducial placement is preferred in order to facilitate robotic SBRT with intra-fraction fiducial tracking for image guidance:

▧ A 4D-CT approach with ITV ± abdominal compression or breath-hold/respiratory gating can also be used.

■ Despite concern for adrenal insufficiency or hypertensive crisis, clinically significant adrenal insufficiency or hypertensive complications after SBRT to the adrenal gland are exceedingly rare. By comparison, IR ablation leads to significantly higher complication rates including adrenal insufficiency and intra-procedural hypertensive crisis (Pan et al. 2020).

Evidence

■ **Meta-analysis of SBRT for adrenal metastases** (Chen et al. 2020): $N = 1006$ patients in 39 retrospective studies with median f/u of 12 months. $N = 63$ patients with bilateral adrenal mets were treated. Median BED-10 was 67 Gy, and median dose was 38 Gy in 5 fx. Pooled 1-year and 2-year LC rates were 82% and 63%, and 1-year and 2-year OS rates were 66% and 42%. A strong relationship between BED-10 and LC was found, and BED-10 of 100 Gy was predicted to correspond to 2-year LC of 85.6% based on meta-regression. Grade 3+ toxicity was 1.8% and was mostly bowel or stomach ulcers and associated bleeds. Only 5 patients (0.5%) were reported to have developed grade 2 adrenal insufficiency, and 1 patient (0.1%) developed hypertensive crisis.

References

Anwar M, Weinberg V, Seymour Z, Hsu IJ, Roach M, Gottschalk AR. Outcomes of hypofractionated stereotactic body radiotherapy boost for intermediate and high-risk prostate cancer. Radiat Oncol. 2016;11(1):8.

Attard G, Murphy L, Clarke N, Cross W, Jones R, Parker C, Gillessen S, Cook A, Brawley C, Amos C, Atako N, Pugh C, Buckner M,

Chowdhury S, Malik Z, Russell J, Gilson C, Rush H, Bowen J, Durr D. Abiraterone acetate and prednisolone with or without enzalutamide for high-risk non-metastatic prostate cancer: a meta-analysis of primary results from two randomised controlled phase 3 trials of the STAMPEDE platform protocol. Lancet. 2022;399(6). https://doi.org/10.1016/S0140-6736(21)02437-5.

Chalkidou A, Macmillan T, Grzeda MT, Peacock J, Summers J, Eddy S, et al. Stereotactic ablative body radiotherapy in patients with oligometastatic cancers: a prospective, registry-based, single-arm, observational, evaluation study. Lancet Oncol. 2021;22(1):98–106.

Chen WC, Baal JD, Baal U, Pai J, Gottschalk A, Boreta L, et al. Stereotactic body radiation therapy of adrenal metastases: a pooled meta-analysis and systematic review of 39 studies with 1006 patients. Int J Radiat Oncol Biol Phys. 2020;107(1):48–61.

Chen WC, Li Y, Lazar A, Altun A, Descovich M, Nano T, et al. Stereotactic body radiation therapy and high-dose-rate brachytherapy boost in combination with intensity modulated radiation therapy for localized prostate cancer: a single-institution propensity score matched analysis. Int J Radiat Oncol Biol Phys. 2021;110(2):429–37. https://www.redjournal.org/article/S0360-3016(20)34730-1/fulltext.

Correa RJM, Louie AV, Zaorsky NG, Lehrer EJ, Ellis R, Ponsky L, et al. The emerging role of stereotactic ablative radiotherapy for primary renal cell carcinoma: a systematic review and meta-analysis. Eur Urol Focus. 2019a;5:958–69.

Correa RJM, Louie AV, Staehler M, Warner A, Gandhidasan S, Ponsky L, et al. Stereotactic radiotherapy as a treatment option for renal tumors in the solitary kidney: a multicenter analysis from the IROCK. J Urol. 2019b;201(6):1097–103.

Cushman TR, Verma V, Khairnar R, Levy J, Simone CB, Mishra MV. Stereotactic body radiation therapy for prostate cancer: systematic review and meta-analysis of prospective trials. Oncotarget. 2019;10(54):5660–8.

D'Agostino G, Franzese C, De Rose F, Franceschini D, Comito T, Villa E, et al. High-quality linac-based stereotactic body radiation therapy with flattening filter free beams and volumetric modulated arc therapy for low–intermediate risk prostate cancer. a mono-institutional experience with 90 patients. Clin Oncol. 2016;28(12):e173–8.

Dang AT, Levin-Epstein RG, Shabsovich D, Cao M, King C, Chu FI, et al. Gantry-mounted linear accelerator–based stereotactic body radiation therapy for low- and intermediate-risk prostate cancer. Adv Radiat Oncol. 2020;5(3):404–11.

De Bleser E, Jereczek-Fossa BA, Pasquier D, Zilli T, Van As N, Siva S, et al. Metastasis-directed therapy in treating nodal Oligorecurrent prostate cancer: a multi-institutional analysis comparing the outcome and toxicity of stereotactic body radiotherapy and elective nodal radiotherapy. Eur Urol. 2019;76(6):732–9.

Gillessen S, Attard G, Beer TM, Beltran H, Bjartell A, Bossi A, et al. Management of Patients with advanced prostate cancer: report of the advanced prostate cancer consensus conference 2019. Eur Urol. 2020;77(4):508–47.

Hall WA, Tree AC, Dearnaley D, Parker CC, Prasad V, Roach M, et al. Considering benefit and risk before routinely recommending SpaceOAR. Lancet Oncol. 2021;22:11–3.

Hofman MS, Lawrentschuk N, Francis RJ, Tang C, Vela I, Thomas P, et al. Prostate-specific membrane antigen PET-CT in patients with high-risk prostate cancer before curative-intent surgery or radiotherapy (proPSMA): a prospective, randomised, multicentre study. Lancet. 2020;395(10231):1208–16.

Jabbari S, Weinberg VK, Kaprealian T, Hsu IC, Ma L, Chuang C, et al. Stereotactic body radiotherapy as monotherapy or post-external beam radiotherapy boost for prostate cancer: technique, early toxicity, and PSA response. Int J Radiat Oncol Biol Phys. 2012;82(1):228–34.

Jackson WC, Silva J, Hartman HE, Dess RT, Kishan AU, Beeler WH, et al. Stereotactic body radiation therapy for localized prostate cancer: a systematic review and meta-analysis of over 6,000 patients treated on prospective studies. Int J Radiat Oncol Biol Phys. 2019;104(4):778–89.

Kaplan ID, Appelbaum L, Aghdam N, Martin J, Sidhom M, Pryor D, Aronovitz JA, Mahadevan A, Kennedy KF, Collins SP. Stereotactic body radiotherapy boost toxicity for high and intermediate-risk prostate cancer: Report of a multi-institutional study. J Clin Oncol. 2020;38(6_suppl):365.

Kim YJ, Ahn H, Kim CS, Kim YS. Phase I/IIa trial of androgen deprivation therapy, external beam radiotherapy, and stereotactic body radiotherapy boost for high-risk prostate cancer (ADEBAR). Radiat Oncol. 2020;15(1):234. https://doi.org/10.1186/s13014-020-01665-6.

Kishan AU, Dang A, Katz AJ, Mantz CA, Collins SP, Aghdam N, et al. Long-term outcomes of stereotactic body radiotherapy for low-risk and intermediate-risk prostate cancer. JAMA Netw Open. 2019;2(2):e188006.

Lehrer EJ, Singh R, Wang M, Chinchilli VM, Trifiletti DM, Ost P, et al. Safety and survival rates associated with ablative stereotactic radiotherapy for patients with oligometastatic cancer: a systematic review and meta-analysis. JAMA Oncol. 2021;7(1):92–106.

Levin-Epstein R, Cook RR, Wong JK, Stock RG, Jeffrey Demanes D, Collins SP, et al. Prostate-specific antigen kinetics and biochemical control following stereotactic body radiation therapy, high dose rate brachytherapy, and low dose rate brachytherapy: a multi-institutional analysis of 3502 patients. Radiother Oncol. 2020;151:26–32.

Meier RM, Bloch DA, Cotrutz C, Beckman AC, Henning GT, Woodhouse SA, et al. Multicenter trial of stereotactic body radiation therapy for low- and intermediate-risk prostate cancer: survival and toxicity endpoints. Int J Radiat Oncol Biol Phys. 2018;102(2):296–303.

Mercado C, Kress MA, Cyr RA, Chen LN, Yung TM, Bullock EG, et al. Intensity-modulated radiation therapy with stereotactic body radiation therapy boost for unfavorable prostate cancer: the Georgetown University experience. Front Oncol. 2016;6:114.

Ost P, Reynders D, Decaestecker K, Fonteyne V, Lumen N, De Bruycker A, et al. Surveillance or metastasis-directed therapy for oligometastatic prostate cancer recurrence (STOMP): five-year results of a randomized phase II trial. J Clin Oncol. 2020;38(6_suppl):10.

Pan S, Baal JD, Chen WC, Baal U, Pai J, Baal J, et al. Image-guided percutaneous ablation of adrenal metastases: a systematic review and meta-analysis. J Vasc Interv Radiol. 2020;32(4):527–535.e1.

Paydar I, Pepin A, Cyr RA, King J, Yung TM, Bullock EG, et al. Intensity-modulated radiation therapy with stereotactic body radiation therapy boost for unfavorable prostate cancer: a report on 3-year toxicity. Front Oncol. 2017;7:5.

Phillips R, Shi WY, Deek M, Radwan N, Lim SJ, Antonarakis ES, et al. Outcomes of observation vs stereotactic ablative radiation for Oligometastatic prostate cancer: the ORIOLE phase 2 randomized clinical trial. JAMA Oncol. 2020;6(5):650–9.

Rosenthal SA, Hu C, Sartor O, Gomella LG, Amin MB, Purdy J, et al. Effect of chemotherapy with docetaxel with androgen suppression and radiotherapy for localized high-risk prostate cancer: the randomized phase III NRG oncology RTOG 0521 trial. J Clin Oncol. 2019;37(14):1159–68.

Siva S, Jackson P, Kron T, Bressel M, Lau E, Hofman M, et al. Impact of stereotactic radiotherapy on kidney function in primary renal cell carcinoma: establishing a dose-response relationship. Radiother Oncol. 2016;118(3):540–6.

Siva S, Bressel M, Murphy DG, Shaw M, Chander S, Violet J, et al. Stereotactic Ablative body radiotherapy (SABR) for Oligometastatic prostate cancer: a prospective clinical trial. Eur Urol. 2018a;74(4):455–62.

Siva S, Louie AV, Warner A, Muacevic A, Gandhidasan S, Ponsky L, et al. Pooled analysis of stereotactic ablative radiotherapy for primary renal cell carcinoma: a report from the international radiosurgery oncology consortium for kidney (IROCK). Cancer. 2018b;124(5):934–42.

Siva S, Correa RJM, Warner A, Staehler M, Ellis RJ, Ponsky L, et al. Stereotactic ablative radiotherapy for ≥T1b primary renal cell carcinoma: a report from the international radiosurgery oncology consortium for kidney (IROCK). Int J Radiat Oncol Biol Phys. 2020;108(4):941–9.

Tree AC, Ostler P, van der Voet H, Chu W, Loblaw A, Ford D, et al. Intensity-modulated radiotherapy versus stereotactic body radiotherapy for prostate cancer (PACE-B): 2-year toxicity results from an open-label, randomised, phase 3, non-inferiority trial. Lancet Oncol. 2022;23(10):1308–20. http://www.ncbi.nlm.nih.gov/pubmed/36113498.

Van As NJ, Brand D, Tree A, Ostler PJ, Chu W, Loblaw A, et al. PACE: analysis of acute toxicity in PACE-B, an international phase III randomized controlled trial comparing stereotactic body radiotherapy (SBRT) to conventionally fractionated or moderately hypofractionated external beam radiotherapy (CFMHRT) for localised prostate cancer. J Clin Oncol. 2019;37(7_suppl):1:1.

Widmark A, Gunnlaugsson A, Beckman L, Thellenberg-Karlsson C, Hoyer M, Lagerlund M, et al. Ultra-hypofractionated versus conventionally fractionated radiotherapy for prostate cancer: 5-year outcomes of the HYPO-RT-PC randomised, non-inferiority, phase 3 trial. Lancet. 2019;394(10196):385–95.

Zaorsky NG, Lehrer EJ, Kothari G, Louie AV, Siva S. Stereotactic ablative radiation therapy for oligometastatic renal cell carcinoma (SABR ORCA): a meta-analysis of 28 studies. Eur Urol Oncol. 2019;2(5):515–23.

Zaorsky NG, Yu JB, McBride SM, Dess RT, Jackson WC, Mahal BA, et al. Prostate cancer radiation therapy recommendations in response to COVID-19. Adv Radiat Oncol. 2020;5(4):659–65.

Zelefsky MJ, Kollmeier M, McBride S, Varghese M, Mychalczak B, Gewanter R, et al. Five-year outcomes of a phase 1 dose-escalation study using stereotactic body radiosurgery for patients with low-risk and intermediate-risk prostate cancer. Int J Radiat Oncol Biol Phys. 2019;104(1):42–9.

Chapter 9
Gynecologic Sites

Matthew S. Susko, Rajni A. Sethi, Zachary A. Seymour, and I-Chow Joe Hsu

Pearls

- SBRT has been employed in recurrent, oligometastatic, and up-front settings for gynecologic tumors, alone or with EBRT.
- There are no randomized trials to evaluate the efficacy and toxicity of SBRT in these settings.
- Local control rate for SBRT re-irradiation of lymph node or distant metastatic sites is ≥65%.

M. S. Susko · I.-C. J. Hsu
Department of Radiation Oncology, University of California, San Francisco, San Francisco, CA, USA
e-mail: Matthew.Susko@ucsf.edu; ihsu@radonc.ucsf.edu; ichow.hsu@ucsf.edu

R. A. Sethi (✉)
Department of Radiation Oncology, Kaiser Permanente, Dublin, CA, USA
e-mail: rajni.a.sethi@kp.org

Z. A. Seymour
Department of Radiation Oncology, Beaumont Health, Sterling Heights, MI, USA
e-mail: Zachary.seymour@beaumont.org

© The Author(s), under exclusive license to Springer Nature Switzerland AG 2023
R. A. Sethi et al. (eds.), *Handbook of Evidence-Based Stereotactic Radiosurgery and Stereotactic Body Radiotherapy*,
https://doi.org/10.1007/978-3-031-33156-5_9

- Local control of small tumors approaches 100% (Choi et al. 2015; Deodato et al. 2009; Guckenberger et al. 2010).
- Local control appears dose dependent with doses $BED_{10} > 70$ for ovarian cancer and possibly higher for other cancers (Macchia et al. 2020; Seo et al. 2015).
- Local control rate for SBRT re-irradiation/pelvic side-wall failures is ~40–50% (Dewas et al. 2011; Park et al. 2015).
- Distant metastasis is the most common failure pattern after SBRT for recurrent tumors with 45–70% 2–4 year distant failure rate.

Treatment Indications

- For gynecologic malignances, SBRT may be indicated to treat isolated lateral pelvic or nodal recurrences or oligometastatic disease (Table 9.1).
- While early studies have explored SBRT techniques to administer a boost dose in definitive radiotherapy for gynecologic malignancies, brachytherapy remains the gold standard for this purpose.
- SBRT should be cautiously utilized for salvage of central recurrences within the high-dose region of the prior treatment field in patients who have undergone definitive radiation owing to its high potential toxicity.

TABLE 9.1 SBRT Treatment Indications

Presentation	Treatment recommendations
Isolated lateral pelvic recurrences	Resection, palliative radiotherapy, or retreatment with SBRT/BT, systemic therapy
Isolated nodal recurrence	Resection, IMRT, re-treatment with SBRT/BT alone, or systemic therapy
Oligometastatic disease	Resection, SBRT/BT, or systemic therapy

Workup and Recommended Imaging

- H&P, including prior radiotherapy, detailed gynecologic history, performance status, pelvic examination.
- Review of systems:
  - Vaginal bleeding.
  - Pelvic or back pain.
  - Neuropathy associated with sidewall recurrences leading to leg pain or weakness.
  - Bowel or bladder symptoms.
- Labs:
  - CBC, metabolic panel, liver function tests.
- Imaging:
  - MRI within 2 weeks of SBRT.
  - PET/CT or CT with contrast as alternatives for recurrent disease.
- Pathology:
  - FNA or CT-guided biopsy of accessible lesions.

Radiosurgical Technique

Simulation and Treatment Planning

- Supine position, arms on chest or overhead.
- Immobilization with body frame and/or fiducial monitoring or bone/body tracking.
- Consider bladder empty or empty and full scan to reproducibly optimize dosimetry to adjacent organs at risk (OARs).
- Thin-cut CT ($\leq$2.5 mm thickness) recommended.
- IV and oral contrast to delineate bowel and vessels.
- GTV is contoured using fusion of the MRI or PET/CT scan merged into the area of interest on simulation CT scan.
- PTV = GTV + 3–8 mm (dependent upon site-specific motion considerations).

- Lower OAR doses can be achieved using a large number of beam angles/arcs and smaller margins.
- Phantom-based QA on all treatment plans prior to delivery of first fraction.

Dose Prescription

- Doses are divided into 1–5 fractions usually over 1–2 weeks.
- SBRT alone in previously unirradiated sites:
  - 6 Gy × 5 fractions (Deodato et al. 2009; Higginson et al. 2011)
  - 11–15 Gy × 3 fractions (Park et al. 2015)
- SBRT alone in previously irradiated fields:
  - 8 Gy × 3 fractions (Kunos et al. 2012)
  - 6 Gy × 5–6 fractions (Deodato et al. 2009; Dewas et al. 2011)
  - 4–5 Gy × 5 fractions (UCSF unpublished)
- SBRT with EBRT 45 Gy for PALN recurrences:
  - 5 Gy × 4–5 fractions (Higginson et al. 2011)
- In series where SBRT has substituted for brachytherapy boost during initial treatment of the primary tumor, dose prescriptions mimic commonly accepted brachytherapy schedules:
  - 7 Gy × 4 fractions (Albuquerque et al. 2020)
- Dose prescribed to 70–80% IDL.

Dose Limitations

- Dose limitations to OAR should meet accepted brachytherapy standards or those as outlined in TG 101 (see Appendix).
- In the setting of re-irradiation, composite planning should be employed, with appropriate BED conversion for dose summation.

Dose Delivery

- Initial verification by kV X-ray or CBCT to visualize the tumor or surrogate markers for positioning.
- Verification imaging should be repeated at least every 5 min for longer treatments.

Toxicities and Management

- Grade 3 or higher acute toxicity or severe late toxicity is rare.
- Common acute toxicities:
  - Fatigue:
    - *Usually self-limiting but* may last for several weeks to months.
  - Urethritis/cystitis:
    - Treatment with phenazopyridine or topical analgesics at the urethral meatus.
  - Dermatitis:
    - Skin erythema, hyperpigmentation, dry desquamation.
    - Limited by increased number of beam angles to reduce entrance and exit doses.
    - Treated with supportive care, including moisturizers, low-dose steroid creams, topical analgesics, and antimicrobial salves.
  - Diarrhea/proctitis:
    - Managed with low-residue diet and antidiarrheals.
  - Nausea:
    - More common with treatment of retroperitoneal nodes leading to bowel dose.
    - Pretreatment with antiemetic 1 h prior to each fraction can limit acute episodes of nausea after treatment.

- Moderate or severe late toxicities:
  - Vaginal stenosis:
    - Managed with vaginal dilator every other day.
  - Ureteral stricture:
    - Expectant management or dilatation procedure.
  - Vesicovaginal or rectovaginal fistula:
    - Surgical management.
  - Intestinal obstruction:
    - Managed with bowel rest or surgical management.
  - Soft-tissue necrosis has been observed particularly in the re-treatment setting. If symptomatic, this may be treated with hyperbaric oxygen therapy.

Recommended Follow-Up

- Pelvic exam every 3 months for 2 years, then every 6 months for 3 years, then annually.
- For cervical cancers, Pap smear every 6 months for 5 years and then annually. Pap smear surveillance should start 6 months after treatment due to postradiation changes.
- PET/CT or CT A/P with contrast 3 months after completion of therapy.

Evidence

SBRT for Oligometastases or as Re-irradiation for Recurrent Tumors

- Kunos et al. (2012): Prospective phase II study, 50 patients with primary gynecologic site, recurrence in ≤4 metastases. Treatment sites were PALN (38%), pelvis (28%), and other distant sites including abdomen, liver, lung, and bone (34%). Dose was 8 Gy × 3 fractions to 70% IDL with Cyberknife. CTV = PET-avid lesions. PTV = CTV + 3 mm. Thirty-two percent had treatment in previously irradiated field. Median follow-up for surviving patients 15 months. No SBRT-treated lesion progressed. Sixty-four percent recurred elsewhere. Three patients (6%) had grade 3–4 toxicity (one grade 3 diarrhea, one enterovaginal fistula, one grade 4 hyperbilirubinemia) (Kunos et al. 2012).

- Dewas et al. (2011): Retrospective study of 16 previously irradiated patients (45 Gy median dose) with pelvic sidewall recurrences. Primary tumors were cervix ($n = 4$), endometrial ($n = 1$), bladder ($n = 1$), anal ($n = 6$), and rectal ($n = 4$). Treatment was 36 Gy to 80% IDL in 6 fractions over 3 weeks with Cyberknife. Median maximum tumor diameter 3.5 cm. 10.6-month median follow-up. One-year actuarial LC 51%. Median DFS 8.3 months. Four of eight patients with sciatic pain had reduction in pain by the end of treatment, but none were able to discontinue opiates. No grade 3 or higher toxicity (Dewas et al. 2011).

- Choi et al. (2009): Retrospective study of 28 cervical cancer patients with isolated PALN metastases. Twenty-four had SBRT 33–45 Gy in 3 fractions; 4 had EBRT followed by SBRT boost. PTV = GTV + 2 mm. Rx to 73–87% IDL. Twenty-five patients received cisplatin-based chemotherapy before ($n = 2$), during ($n = 9$), or after ($n = 14$) SBRT. Four-year LC was 68% overall, and 100% if PTV volume ≤17 mL (Choi et al. 2009).

- Higginson et al. (2011): Retrospective study of 16 patients treated with SBRT (9 recurrences, 5 SBRT boost, 2 oligometastatic). SBRT doses were 12–54 Gy in 3–5 fractions. Eleven patients had additional EBRT 30–54 Gy. Eleven-month median follow-up. LC 79%. Distant failure 43% (Higginson et al. 2011).

- Guckenberger et al. (2010): Retrospective study of 19 patients with isolated pelvic recurrence after primary surgical treatment (12 cervix, 7 endometrial primaries). Sixteen previously unirradiated cases had 50 Gy EBRT followed by SBRT boost; 3 patients with prior

RT had SBRT alone. Patients were selected for SBRT over brachytherapy due to size (>4.5 cm) and/or peripheral location. Dose for SBRT boost was 5 Gy × 3 fractions to median 65% IDL; SBRT only 10 Gy × 3 fractions or 7 Gy × 4 fractions to the 65% IDL. Three-year LC 81%. Median time to systemic progression 16 months. Sixteen percent severe complication rate (2 intestino-vaginal fistulas and one small bowel ileus). Two of the patients with severe complications had prior pelvic RT ± brachytherapy and had bowel maximum point dose of EQD2 >80 Gy (Guckenberger et al. 2010).

- Deodato et al. (2009): Retrospective study of 11 patients, dose escalation with 5 daily SBRT fractions up to 6 Gy per fraction, in previously irradiated ($n = 6$) or previously unirradiated ($n = 5$) patients with recurrent gynecologic tumors. Two-year local PFS 82%. Two-year DMFS 54%. No grade 3–4 toxicity (Deodato et al. 2009).
- Seo et al. (2015): Retrospective review of 88 patients with para-aortic recurrences treated with SBRT, of which 52 were from primary gynecological sites and 36 were from other sites. $BED_{10} \geq 95$ Gy ($p = 0.011$) and gross tumor volume (GTV) ≤ 15 cm^3 ($p = 0.002$) were associated with better local control (Seo et al. 2015).
- Park et al. (2015): Retrospective multi-institutional (KROG 14–11) cohort of 85 patients and 100 lesions treated with SBRT for recurrent or oligometastatic uterine cancer. Predominantly (89%) lymph node metastases, with 59 within the prior radiation field, treated to a median dose of 39 Gy in 3 fractions (BED_{10} 90 Gy). Overall, 2 and 5-year LC rates were 82.5% and 78.8%, with OS at 2 and 5 years of 57.5% and 32.9%, respectively, and only 5 incidence of grade 3+ toxicity. 2-Year local control was worse for lesions within a previously irradiated field (60.2% vs. 92.8%, $p < 0.01$) and tended to marginally become better for lesions treated with $BED_{10} \geq 69.3$ Gy (87.7% vs. 66.1%

$p < 0.59$) of which previously irradiated tumors had lower marginal doses (Park et al. 2015).

- Macchia et al. (2020): Retrospective multi-institution (MITO RT-01) study of 261 ovarian cancer patients with metastatic, recurrent, or persistent disease treated with SBRT. Inclusive of any anatomic site, median BED_{10} of 50.7 Gy (range: 7.5–262.5) with a median of 1 lesion (range: 1–7) treated. At a median follow-up of 22 months, 2-year LC was 81.9%, with 95.1% late toxicity-free survival at 2 years. On MVA, patient age ≤60 years (OR 1.6), PTV volume ≤18 cm^3 (OR 1.9), lymph node treatment site (OR 2.9), and $BED_{10} > 70$ Gy (OR 2.0) were associated with improved rates of complete response (Macchia et al. 2020).

- Yegya-Raman et al. (2020): Meta-analysis of 17 studies and 667 patients with 1071 metastatic lesions from gynecologic malignancies. Predominantly ovarian (57.6%), cervical (27.1%), and uterine (11.1%), with most patients having a single metastatic site (65.4%). Response rate ranged from 49 to 97%, with most (7/8 studies) reporting >75% response. Crude local control ranged from 71 to 100% with most (14/16 studies) demonstrating a local control of >80%. Grade ≥3 toxicities were not observed in 10/16 studies. Those studies reporting grade ≥3 toxicity observed this in 2.6–10% of patients. SBRT was well tolerated with high rates of efficacy, with disease progression most commonly being reported at a distant site (79–100%) (Yegya-Raman et al. 2020).

SBRT Boost in Initial Definitive Radiotherapy

- Kemmerer et al. (2013): Retrospective study of 11 patients with stage I–III endometrial cancer. Definitive EBRT 45 Gy followed by SBRT boost to the high-risk CTV (1 cm around endometrium and any gross disease after EBRT). Dose: 30 Gy/5 fractions in nine patients, 20–24 Gy/4 fractions in two patients, and two fractions/week. IMRT-based treatment with daily kV CBCT. Ten-month median follow-up. One-year FFP of 68% for all patients, 2-year FFP 100% for grade 1 or stage IA tumors. Eighty percent of failures were in endometrium. One grade 3 toxicity (diarrhea) (Kemmerer et al. 2013).

- Mollà et al. (2005): Retrospective study of 16 patients with endometrial ($n = 9$) or cervical ($n = 7$) cancer treated with SBRT boost, 7 Gy × 2 (post-op, $n = 12$) or 4 Gy × 5 (no surgery, $n = 4$), two SBRT fractions per week. PTV = CTV + 6–10 mm. Median follow-up 12.6 months. Dynamic arc therapy or IMRT was used. Only 1 failure in a cervix cancer patient. One patient had grade 3 rectal toxicity (persistent rectal bleeding) and was treated previously with pelvic RT with HDR boost (Mollà et al. 2005).

- Marnitz et al. (2013): Retrospective review of 11 patients with cervical cancer treated with SBRT boost 6 Gy × 5 fractions to 60–70% IDL QOD. PTV coverage was 93–99% to meet constraints. No grade 3 toxicity reported (Marnitz et al. 2013).

- Mantz et al. (2016): Prospective phase II trial of curative-intent SBRT boost for patients with uterine or cervical cancer unable or unwilling to undergo surgery or brachytherapy boost. Excluded patients with GTV >125 cc. Primary definitive treatment to the pelvis of 45 Gy in 25-fraction EBRT followed by boost to the GTV of 40 Gy in 5-fraction EOD. Target was tumor plus PTV margin, and delineation of the GTV was aided by co-registration of FDG-PET imaging to the CT planning image set. Overall, 40 patients were enrolled with a median follow-up of 51 months, 33/40 (82.5%) had negative post-SBRT biopsy for invasive malignancy, and 2-year post-SBRT FDG-PET showed complete response at the primary site of disease in 77.5% of patients. No reported incidence of grade ≥3 toxicity was noted (Mantz et al. 2015).

- Albuquerque et al. (2020): Single-arm prospective phase II trial of SBRT boost for FIGO 2009 stage IB2–IVB cervical cancer, medically unfit to undergo brachytherapy boost, treated with SBRT to 28 Gy in 4 fractions >36 h apart. CTV volume was larger than prior reports, including T2-MR gross tumor, cervix, at least 2 cm of the normal uterine canal with PTV margin 0.3 cm axial and 0.5 cm longitudinal. Overall, 15 patients accrued (53% stage III–IV), with a median follow-up of 19 months. Median SBRT boost volume was 139 cc (range: 51–268), 2-year local control 70.1%, PFS 46.7%, and OS 53.3%, all lower than expected. Smaller PTV boost in patients without grade ≥ 3 (95 cc versus 225 cc). Patients experiencing grade 3 toxicity were 26.7%, and dosimetric analysis demonstrated that the percentage of rectal circumference receiving 15 Gy was associated with V15 Gy ($p = 0.04$) with volumes >62.7% being the strongest predictor of toxicity (AUC, 0.93; sensitivity, 100%; specificity, 90%) (Albuquerque et al. 2020).

References

Albuquerque K, Tumati V, Lea J, Ahn C, Richardson D, Miller D, et al. A phase II trial of stereotactic ablative radiation therapy as a boost for locally advanced cervical cancer. Int J Radiat Oncol Biol Phys. 2020;106(3):464–71.

Choi CW, Cho CK, Yoo SY, Kim MS, Yang KM, Yoo HJ, et al. Image-guided stereotactic body radiation therapy in patients with isolated Para-aortic lymph node metastases from uterine cervical and corpus cancer. Int J Radiat Oncol Biol Phys. 2009;74(1):147–53.

Choi JW, Im YS, Kong DS, Seol HJ, Nam DH, Il LJ. Effectiveness of postoperative gamma knife radiosurgery to the tumor bed after resection of brain metastases. World Neurosurg. 2015;84(6):1752–7.

Deodato F, Macchia G, Grimaldi L, Ferrandina G, Lorusso D, Salutari V, et al. Stereotactic radiotherapy in recurrent gynecological cancer: a case series. Oncol Rep. 2009;22(2):415–9.

Dewas S, Bibault JE, Mirabel X, Nickers P, Castelain B, Lacornerie T, et al. Robotic image-guided reirradiation of lateral pelvic recurrences: preliminary results. Radiat Oncol. 2011;6(1):77.

Guckenberger M, Bachmann J, Wulf J, Mueller G, Krieger T, Baier K, et al. Stereotactic body radiotherapy for local boost irradiation in unfavourable locally recurrent gynaecological cancer. Radiother Oncol. 2010;94(1):53–9.

Higginson DS, Morris DE, Jones EL, Clarke-Pearson D, Varia MA. Stereotactic body radiotherapy (SBRT): technological innovation and application in gynecologic oncology. Gynecol Oncol. 2011;120(3):404–12.

Kemmerer E, Hernandez E, Ferriss JS, Valakh V, Miyamoto C, Li S, et al. Use of image-guided stereotactic body radiation therapy in lieu of intracavitary brachytherapy for the treatment of inoperable endometrial neoplasia. Int J Radiat Oncol Biol Phys. 2013;85(1):129–35.

Kunos CA, Brindle J, Waggoner S, Zanotti K, Resnick K, Fusco N, et al. Phase II clinical trial of robotic stereotactic body radiosurgery for metastatic gynecologic malignancies. Front. Oncologia. 2012;2:2.

Macchia G, Lazzari R, Colombo N, Laliscia C, Capelli G, D'Agostino GR, et al. A large, multicenter, retrospective study on efficacy and safety of stereotactic body radiotherapy (SBRT) in Oligometastatic ovarian cancer (MITO RT1 study): a collaboration of MITO, AIRO GYN, and MaNGO groups. Oncologist. 2020;25(2):e311–20.

Mantz CA, Shahin FA, Sandadi S, Orr J. Stereotactic body radiation therapy as a boost alternative to brachytherapy for primary gynecologic cancer: disease control and quality of life outcomes from a phase II trial. Int J Radiat Oncol. 2015;93(3):S202.

Marnitz S, Kohler C, Budach V, Neumann O, Kluge A, Wlodarczyk W, Jhan U, Debauer B, Kufeld M. Brachytherapy-emulating robotic radiosurgery in patients with cervical carcinoma. Radiat Oncol. 2013;8:109.

Mollà M, Escude L, Nouet P, Popowski Y, Hidalgo A, Rouzaud M, et al. Fractionated stereotactic radiotherapy boost for gynecologic tumors: an alternative to brachytherapy? Int J Radiat Oncol Biol Phys. 2005;62(1):118–24.

Park HJ, Chang AR, Seo Y, Cho CK, Il JW, Kim MS, et al. Stereotactic body radiotherapy for recurrent or oligometastatic uterine cervix cancer: a cooperative study of the Korean radiation oncology group (KROG 14-11). Anticancer Res. 2015;35(9):5103–10.

Seo YS, Kim MS, Cho CK, Yoo HH, Jang WI, Kim KB, Lee DH, Moon SM, Lee HR. Stereotactic body radiotherapy for oligometastases confined to the Para-aortic region: clinical outcomes and the significance of radiotherapy field and dose. Cancer Investig. 2015;33(5):18–7.

Yegya-Raman N, Cao CD, Hathout L, Girda E, Richard SD, Rosenblum NG, et al. Stereotactic body radiation therapy for oligometastatic gynecologic malignancies: a systematic review. Gynecol Oncol. 2020;159:573–80.

Chapter 10
Soft Tissue Sarcoma

Katherine S. Chen, Steve E. Braunstein, and Alexander R. Gottschalk

Pearls

- ~13,500 cases/year and ~5400 deaths/year in the USA (American Cancer Society 2021).
- Staging is classified by anatomic site: extremity/trunk (~55%), retroperitoneal (~15%), head and neck (~10%), and visceral sites (~20%) (National Comprehensive Cancer Network 2021).
- Associated with genetic predisposition syndromes: NF-1, retinoblastoma, Gardner syndrome, Li-Fraumeni syndrome.
- Limb-sparing surgery combined with pre- or postoperative radiotherapy is the current standard of care for extremity STS with LC >90% (O'Sullivan et al. 2002).
- Especially with high-grade large primary tumors, up to 25–40% of patients may develop distant metastasis, most commonly to lung, followed by bone, liver, and brain (Zagars et al. 2003).

K. S. Chen (✉) · S. E. Braunstein · A. R. Gottschalk
Department of Radiation Oncology, University of California, San Francisco, San Francisco, CA, USA
e-mail: Katherine.chen5@ucsf.edu; Steve.Braunstein@ucsf.edu; Alexander.Gottschalk@ucsf.edu

© The Author(s), under exclusive license to Springer Nature Switzerland AG 2023
R. A. Sethi et al. (eds.), *Handbook of Evidence-Based Stereotactic Radiosurgery and Stereotactic Body Radiotherapy*,
https://doi.org/10.1007/978-3-031-33156-5_10

- Several STS histologies have been associated with lower α/β ratio, suggesting an effective response with hypofractionation, which has been demonstrated in several studies of SBRT and SRS of lung, brain, and spinal STS metastases (van Leeuwen et al. 2018).
- Common neoadjuvant/adjuvant systemic therapy options include doxorubicin and ifosfamide, gemcitabine and docetaxel for less medically fit or older patients aged >65, and imatinib for c-kit GIST.
- Metastatic STS is associated with poor median survival ~1 year, but treatment of oligometastatic disease is associated with improved survival (Gronchi et al. 2016).

Workup and Recommended Imaging

- H&P, CBC, BUN/Cr, ESR, LDH, plain X-ray films of primary.
- CT/MRI for treatment planning and assessment of peritumoral edema.
- Biopsy for primary (core needle biopsy preferred; incisional biopsy may be considered by an experienced surgeon).
- Biopsy for suspected metastatic disease should be considered for the confirmation of oligometastatic disease but is otherwise generally avoided in patients with previously biopsy-proven disease due to concern for further disease seeding.

Treatment Indications

- Preoperative and/or postoperative EBRT +/− IORT used in primary setting.
- SBRT generally not recommended preoperatively due to historically large margin recommendations for extremity STS (3–5 cm longitudinal and 1–2 cm circumferential), although studies are investigating the role of hypofractionated treatment in the preoperative setting.

- Potential role for SBRT as small-volume postoperative boost following preoperative EBRT and resection with positive margins.
- SBRT may be used in recurrent or metastatic disease for symptomatic palliation. SBRT should be strongly considered for patients with oligometastatic disease who are poor surgical candidates due to comorbidities or resectability concerns (Table 10.1).

TABLE 10.1 Treatment paradigm for STS

Disease site	Presentation	Recommended treatment
Extremity	Early stage (I) Intermediate-advanced stage (II–III)	Surgery → EBRT for +/− close margin Surgery → post-op EBRT or pre-op EBRT → surgery, +/− chemo for deep/high-grade tumors
Retroperitoneal	Resectable	Surgery + IORT → post-op EBRT or pre-op EBRT → surgery + IORT
GIST	Resectable Unresectable	Surgery +/− imatinib Imatinib → re-eval +/− surgery
Desmoid	Asymptomatic Resectable Unresectable	Consider observation Surgery +/− EBRT for +margin or definitive EBRT or systemic therapy EBRT, systemic therapy
Metastatic (stage IV)	Chest, abdominal, or pelvic oligometastases Spinal metastases Diffuse metastases	Surgical metastasectomy, SBRT, systemic therapy Surgical resection/ stabilization, EBRT/ SBRT Systemic therapy, EBRT/ SBRT for palliation of selected involved sites

Radiosurgical Technique

- Dose and fractionation directed by adjacent normal tissue RT toxicity constraints.

Simulation and Treatment Planning

- If biopsy or resection is performed, request fiducial marker placement.
- Prefer fine-cut (1–1.5 mm) treatment planning CT ± contrast with 4DCT to define ITV for thoracic or upper abdominal metastases.
- Immobilization with body frame and/or fiducial, lesion, or vertebral element tracking.
- Abdominal compression and/or respiratory gating may be employed to reduce lesion motion associated with diaphragmatic excursion during breathing.
- Image fusion with diagnostic CT, MRI, myelogram, and/or PET for target delineation as appropriate.
- GTV/iGTV = lesion as defined by CT or MRI-based imaging, with contrast as available. Lung windowing should be used for pulmonary oligometastases.
- CTV/ITV = GTV/iGTV + 0–10 mm (CTV/ITV = GTV/iGTV for pulmonary lesions).
- PTV = CTV/ITV + 3–5 mm (smaller margins with intrafraction image guidance and/or motion management).
- Image guidance with orthogonal kV and/or cone beam CT for daily treatment delivery.

Dose Prescription

- Peripheral lung oligometastases:
  - 25–34 Gy × 1 fx, 18 Gy × 3 fx, 12 Gy × 4 fx, 10 Gy × 5 fx
- Central and ultra-central lung oligometastases:
  - 10 Gy × 5 fx, 7.5 Gy × 8 fx, 4 Gy × 15 fx

- Abdominal and pelvic oligometastases:
  - 6–8 Gy × 5 fx
- Vertebral spine metastases:
  - 18–24 Gy × 1 fx, 8–10 Gy × 3 fx, 6–8 Gy × 5 fx

Toxicities and Management

- EBRT late radiation morbidities include decreased range of motion secondary to fibrosis at primary site, lymphedema with circumferential treatment of extremities, and low risk of secondary malignancy. Postoperative wound healing complications are higher with preoperative radiation as compared to postoperative radiation (O'Sullivan et al. 2002; Davis et al. 2005).
- SBRT toxicity related to dose and volume of treated adjacent normal tissues.
  - Risk of skin toxicity and bone fracture for tumors located in the extremity.
  - Risk of lung injury for pulmonary metastases (see corresponding chapter).
  - Risk of liver, adrenal, renal, and bowel toxicity for abdominal metastases. Nausea most common acute toxicity for abdominal SBRT, often responsive to short-term antiemetic pharmacotherapy.
  - Acute pain flare, vertebral insufficiency fracture, and risk of late myelopathy for spinal metastases.

Recommended Follow-Up

- Exam with functional status, MRI of primary, CT chest every 3 months × 2 years, then every 4 months × 1 year, and then every 6 months × 2 years.
- CT imaging of treated oligometastatic site every 3 months × 1 year.
- Consider bone scan, MRI, or PET, if clinically indicated.

Evidence

- There is a lack of randomized prospective data on the use of SBRT approaches in primary, recurrent, and metastatic disease.

Primary STS

- While there is limited data regarding SBRT in the management of primary STS, there is evidence of efficacy of short-course hypofractionated RT in both the preoperative and postoperative settings, delivered via EBRT, SBRT, or brachytherapy. Major wound complications and late toxicity with hypofractionated regimens appear comparable to conventionally fractionated courses.
- Studies have also shown improved outcomes with reduced treatment-volume IGRT and IMRT techniques, which may also allow for dose escalation:
  - Wang et al. (2015): Multi-institutional phase II study of reduced target volumes with preoperative IGRT (75% IMRT, 25% 3DCRT) for 79 patients with extremity STS showed significant reduction in grade 2+ late toxicity when compared to historical controls (11% vs. 37%, $p < 0.001$). Five patients with LR, most with +margins and all within CTV as opposed to marginal failure.
  - Folkert et al. (2019): Retrospective series of 92 patients with primary STS of the thigh/groin demonstrated lower than expected risk of femoral fracture (7% vs. 26% as calculated by Princess Margaret Hospital nomogram) with the use of perioperative IMRT (14% preoperative, 86% postoperative) for increased bone sparing as compared to 3DCRT.

Preoperative Radiation

- Koseła-Paterczyk et al. (2014): Prospective study of 272 patients with extremity/trunk STS treated with hypofractionated preoperative 3DCRT (25 Gy in 5 fx), followed by immediate surgery. LR 19% at a median follow-up of 35 months, 3-year OS 72%. Acute toxicity in 32%, and late toxicity in 15%. Seven percent required additional surgery for wound complications.
- Pennington et al. (2018): Retrospective series of 116 patients with extremity STS treated with neoadjuvant ifosfamide-based chemotherapy and hypofractionated preoperative 3DCRT (28 Gy in 8 fx), followed by surgery 1–2 weeks later. LR 11% and OS 82% at 3 years. LR 17% and OS 67% at 6 years. Ten percent with acute/perioperative complications.
- Kubicek et al. (2018): Phase II study of 13 patients with extremity STS treated with preoperative SBRT (35–40 Gy in 5 fx, all on CyberKnife with fiducials), followed by surgery 4–8 weeks later. All patients had R0 resections. One patient developed LR at 16 months. Four patients underwent planned vacuum-assisted wound closures, but there were no other major wound complications.
- Koseła-Paterczyk et al. (2020): Phase II study of 29 patients with myxoid liposarcoma of the lower limb treated with hypofractionated preoperative RT (25 Gy in 5 fx, 38% IMRT with remainder 3DCRT), followed by surgery at a median of 7 weeks later. LC 100% at a median follow-up of 27 months. Acute toxicity in 38%, and late toxicity in 14%. Wound complications in 38%.
- Kalbasi et al. (2020): Phase II study of 52 patients with extremity/trunk STS treated with hypofraction-

ated preoperative RT (30 Gy in 5 fx, 76% IMRT with remainder 3DCRT/electrons), followed by surgery 2–6 weeks later. Two-year LR 6%, and OS 84%. Major wound complications in 32%.

Postoperative Radiation

- Itami et al. (2010): Retrospective series of 25 primary STS patients treated postoperatively with HDR monotherapy, 36 Gy in 6 fx in 3 days b.i.d. LC 78% at 5 years, but up to 93% for patients with negative margins and no prior surgical resections. Late grade 2+ wound toxicity 12%.
- Petera et al. (2010): Retrospective series of 45 primary or recurrent STS patients treated postoperatively with HDR monotherapy (30–54 Gy, 3 Gy b.i.d. fx) vs. HDR (15–30 Gy, 3 Gy b.i.d. fx) + EBRT (40–50 Gy at 1.8–2 Gy fx). LC 74% and OS 70% at 5 years. LC better for primary tumors (100%) and for patients treated with combination HDR + EBRT vs. HDR monotherapy (OR 0.2, $p = 0.04$).
- Naghavi et al. (2017): Consensus guidelines for brachytherapy for soft tissue sarcoma recommend consideration of brachytherapy monotherapy for small high-grade tumors, re-irradiation, frail and elderly patients, or children. Combination HDR and EBRT may be used for large tumors, recurrent disease, or close margins.
- Soyfer et al. (2013): Series of 21 elderly patients with median age 80 treated with postoperative hypofractionated EBRT, 39–48 Gy in 13–16 fx. LC 86% at a median follow-up of 26 months. Three patients had LR, all with <3 mm surgical margins. Three patients noted with late grade 2–3 toxicity.

Metastatic STS

Surgical or Radiofrequency Ablation

- Potential survival benefit for ablative treatment of oligometastatic disease suggested by multiple surgical series.
- Billingsley et al. (1999): Retrospective series of 719 patients with STS pulmonary metastases. MS 33 months for patients receiving complete metastasectomy vs. 11 months for those receiving nonoperative therapy.
- Porter et al. (2004): Comparative effectiveness study of surgical metastasectomy vs. systemic chemotherapy for the treatment of pulmonary STS metastases. Despite favorable assumptions of benefit of chemotherapy, surgical ablative therapy was deemed a significantly more cost-effective management approach.
- Chudgar et al. (2017): Retrospective review of 539 patients with STS pulmonary metastases. MS 33 months. Factors associated with better OS included leiomyosarcoma histology, smaller primary tumor size, longer interval from resection of primary to development of metastasis, solitary lung metastasis, and minimally invasive resection.
- DeMatteo et al. (2001): Retrospective series of 331 patients treated for STS liver metastases, of which 56 patients underwent R0 or R1 gross resection of hepatic metastases. MS 39 months vs. 12 months for those who did not undergo complete or any resection independent of adjuvant systemic therapy.
- Pawlik et al. (2006): Retrospective series of 66 patients who underwent hepatic resection and/or RFA of STS liver metastases. OS 91% at 1 year, 65% at 3 years, and 27% at 5 years. Increased risk of local recurrence in

patients who underwent RFA +/− resection compared to resection alone (85–89% vs. 57%, $p < 0.05$).

- Marudanayagam et al. (2011): Retrospective series of 36 patients who underwent hepatic resection for oligometastatic STS. OS 90% at 1 year, 48% at 3 years, and 32% at 5 years. Poor survival associated with high-grade tumors, primary leiomyosarcoma, and positive resection margin of liver metastasis.

Radiotherapy for Metastatic Disease

- Studies have shown excellent rates of local control and minimal toxicity with SBRT/SRS for STS metastases in lung, spine, liver, and brain. Emerging non-randomized evidence suggests that local therapy for oligometastatic STS in particular may delay the course of disease or even lead to potential survival benefit.
- Falk et al. (2015): Retrospective series of 281 patients with 1–5 STS oligometastases treated with local ablative therapies (including surgery, RFA, RT). Improved MS of 45 months in those receiving local treatment vs. 13 months in those without.
- Savina et al. (2017): Large observational study of 2165 patients with metastatic STS showed prolonged time to next treatment and improved overall survival in patients who received locoregional treatment for metastases (including surgery, RFA, RT).

SBRT for Lung Metastases

- Corbin et al. (2007): Retrospective series of 58 patients with STS pulmonary metastases. Sixteen patients received SBRT to a median of 4.5 nodules. OS 73% at 2.5 years for SBRT patients vs. 25% for the remaining

42 patients treated with EBRT, surgery, and/or chemotherapy. SBRT found associated with improved outcome on both univariate (HR = 0.43, p = 0.012) and multivariate analyses (p = 0.007).

- Dhakal et al. (2012): Retrospective series of 15 patients treated with SBRT to 74 lesions for STS pulmonary metastases with preferred dose of 50 Gy in 5 fx. LC 82% at 3 years. No grade 3+ toxicity. MS 2.1 years vs. 0.6 years for 37 patients not receiving SBRT for pulmonary STS metastases (p = 0.002).
- Mehta et al. (2013): Retrospective series of 16 patients treated with SBRT to 25 lesions for high-grade STS lung metastases. Prescription dose ranged from 36 to 54 Gy in 3–4 fx. LC 94% at 43 months. No grade 2+ pneumonitis or esophagitis.
- Soyfer et al. (2017): Retrospective series of 22 patients with 53 STS pulmonary metastases treated with SBRT (mostly 60 Gy in 3 fx). SBRT was able to control 100% of lesions measuring <1 cm vs. 72% of lesions >1 cm in size, although no treated lesions ultimately progressed at a median follow-up of 94 months. Of lesions <1 cm, 71% achieved complete response at median 6 months. OS 62% at 5 years.
- Lindsay et al. (2018): Retrospective series of 44 patients with 117 pulmonary metastases from sarcoma treated with SBRT (mostly 50 Gy in 10 fx). LC 95% and OS 50% at 5 years. Eleven patients with radiation-associated complications, including 6 patients with grade 1–3 pneumonitis and 1 patient with grade 4 esophageal stricture.
- Baumann et al. (2020): Multi-institutional series of 44 patients with 56 pulmonary metastases from sarcoma treated with SBRT (typically 50 Gy in 4–5 fx). OS 74% at 1 year and 46% at 2 years. LC 96% at 1 year and 90% at 2 years. No grade 3+ toxicities.

SBRT for Spine Metastases

- Levine et al. (2009): Retrospective series of ten patients with primary and metastatic spinal sarcomas treated with palliative-intent SBRT (median dose 30 Gy in 3 fx). Patients experienced complete pain relief in 50%, partial relief in 44%, and no relief in 6% of treated lesions. MS 11 months from the time of SBRT.
- Folkert et al. (2014) and Leeman et al. (2016): Retrospective series of 88 patients with 120 sarcoma-related (predominantly STS) spinal metastases. Patients received multifraction (24–36 Gy in 3–6 fx) or single-fraction (18–24 Gy) SBRT. OS 61% at 1 year. One percent acute and 4.5% chronic grade 3 toxicity. Single-fraction was superior to multifraction SBRT, with LC rates of 91% vs. 84%, respectively ($p = 0.007$). Overall, freedom from failure within the spine was 58% at 1 year. On patterns of failure analysis, the majority had distant failures (≥ 2 segments from the treated lesion), with only 7% experiencing an isolated local or adjacent-level failure.
- Miller et al. (2017): Retrospective series of 18 patients with 40 primary and metastatic sarcoma spine lesions treated with SBRT (median dose 16 Gy in 1 fx). Pain relief in 82% at 6 months, with median time to pain progression of 10 months. Radiographic failure in 48% at median 14 months. MS 16 months after SBRT.
- Bishop et al. (2017): Retrospective series of 48 patients with 66 spinal metastases from sarcoma treated with SBRT (47% single fraction). LC 81% and OS 67% at 1 year. BED ≤ 48 Gy and postoperative setting associated with worse local control ($p = 0.006$, $p = 0.06$). Among 14 cases of local recurrence, 10 were within the epidural space and 4 were in the paraspinal musculature. Four patients with late insufficiency fractures.

SBRT for Liver Metastases

■ Kollar et al. (2015): Retrospective series including 10 patients with 19 liver metastases from sarcoma treated with SBRT (median 50 Gy in 5 fx). No lesions progressed at a median follow-up of 10 months, and 63% showed complete or partial response. Median chemotherapy-free holiday of 6.5 months.

SRS for Brain Metastases

■ Chang et al. (2005): Retrospective series of 189 patients treated with SRS for "radioresistant" histologies of brain metastasis, including melanoma (103), RCC (77), and sarcoma (9). Median single-session SRS dose was 18 Gy (10–24 Gy), prescribed by tumor size based upon RTOG 90-05 guidelines. Among patients with sarcoma metastases, MS was 9.1 months at a median follow-up.

■ Sim et al. (2020): Retrospective series of 24 patients with 58 STS brain metastases treated with LINAC-based SRS/FSRT. LC 89% and OS 38% at 1 year. All four lesions that failed locally were of primary spindle cell histology.

References

American Cancer Society. Cancer facts and figures. 2021. https://www.cancer.org/content/dam/cancer-org/research/cancer-facts-and-statistics/annual-cancer-facts-and-figures/2021/cancer-facts-and-figures-2021.pdf. Accessed 18 Mar 2021.

Baumann BC, Bernstein KDA, DeLaney TF, Simone CB, Kolker JD, Choy E, et al. Multi-institutional analysis of stereotactic body radiotherapy for sarcoma pulmonary metastases: high rates of local control with favorable toxicity. J Surg Oncol. 2020;122(5):877–83.

Billingsley KG, Burt ME, Jara E, Ginsberg RJ, Woodruff JM, Leung DHY, et al. Pulmonary metastases from soft tissue sarcoma: analysis of patterns of disease and postmetastasis survival. Ann Surg. 1999;229(5):602–12.

Bishop AJ, Tao R, Guadagnolo BA, Allen PK, Rebueno NC, Wang XA, et al. Spine stereotactic radiosurgery for metastatic sarcoma: patterns of failure and radiation treatment volume considerations. J Neurosurg Spine. 2017;27(3):303–11.

Chang EL, Selek U, Hassenbusch SJ, Maor MH, Allen PK, Mahajan A, et al. Outcome variation among "radioresistant" brain metastases treated with stereotactic radiosurgery. Neurosurgery. 2005;56(5):936–44.

Chudgar NP, Brennan MF, Munhoz RR, Bucciarelli PR, Tan KS, D'Angelo SP, et al. Pulmonary metastasectomy with therapeutic intent for soft-tissue sarcoma. J Thorac Cardiovasc Surg. 2017;154(1):319–330.e1. https://doi.org/10.1016/j.jtcvs.2017.02.061.

Corbin K, Philip A, Hyrien O, Saharsrabudhe D, Chen R, Jones C, et al. Do patients with pulmonary metastases from soft tissue sarcoma benefit from stereotactic body radiation therapy. Int J Radiat Oncol Biol Phys. 2007;69(3):S752.

Davis AM, O'Sullivan B, Turcotte R, Bell R, Catton C, Chabot P, et al. Late radiation morbidity following randomization to preoperative versus postoperative radiotherapy in extremity soft tissue sarcoma. Radiother Oncol. 2005;75(1):48–53.

DeMatteo R, Shah A, Fong Y. Results of hepatic resection for sarcoma metastatic to liver. Ann Surg. 2001;234(4):540–8. http://www.ncbi.nlm.nih.gov/pmc/articles/pmc1422077/.

Dhakal S, Corbin KS, Milano MT, Philip A, Sahasrabudhe D, Jones C, et al. Stereotactic body radiotherapy for pulmonary metastases from soft-tissue sarcomas: excellent local lesion control and improved patient survival. Int J Radiat Oncol Biol Phys. 2012;82(2):940–5.

Falk AT, Moureau-Zabotto L, Ouali M, Penel N, Italiano A, Bay JO, et al. Effect on survival of local ablative treatment of metastases from sarcomas: a study of the French sarcoma group. Clin Oncol. 2015;27(1):48–55. https://doi.org/10.1016/j.clon.2014.09.010.

Folkert MR, Bilsky MH, Tom AK, Oh JH, Alektiar KM, Laufer I, et al. Outcomes and toxicity for hypofractionated and single-fraction image-guided stereotactic radiosurgery for sarcomas metastasizing to the spine. Int J Radiat Oncol Biol Phys. 2014;88(5):1085–91.

Folkert MR, Casey DL, Berry SL, Crago A, Fabbri N, Singer S, et al. Femoral fracture in primary soft-tissue sarcoma of the thigh and groin treated with intensity-modulated radiation therapy: observed versus expected risk. Ann Surg Oncol. 2019;26(5):1326–31. https://doi.org/10.1245/s10434-019-07182-5.

Gronchi A, Guadagnolo BA, Erinjeri JP. Local ablative therapies to metastatic soft tissue sarcoma. Am Soc Clin Oncol Educ B. 2016;36:e566–75.

Itami J, Sumi M, Beppu Y, Chuman H, Kawai A, Murakami N, et al. High-dose rate brachytherapy alone in postoperative soft tissue sarcomas with close or positive margins. Brachytherapy. 2010;9(4):349–53.

Kalbasi A, Kamrava M, Chu FI, Telesca D, Van Dams R, Yang Y, et al. A phase II trial of 5-day neoadjuvant radiotherapy for patients with high-risk primary soft tissue sarcoma. Clin Cancer Res. 2020;26(8):1829–36.

Kollar LE, Sapir E, Welling TH, Chugh R, Schuetze SM, Lawrence TS, et al. Local management for sarcoma liver metastases. Int J Radiat Oncol. 2015;93(3):E633. https://doi.org/10.1016/j.ijrobp.2015.07.2163.

Koseła-Paterczyk H, Szacht M, Morysiński T, Ługowska I, Dziewirski W, Falkowski S, et al. Preoperative hypofractionated radiotherapy in the treatment of localized soft tissue sarcomas. Eur J Surg Oncol. 2014;40(12):1641–7.

Koseła-Paterczyk H, Spałek M, Borkowska A, Teterycz P, Wągrodzki M, Szumera-Ciećkiewicz A, et al. Hypofractionated radiotherapy in locally advanced Myxoid Liposarcomas of extremities or trunk wall: results of a single-arm prospective clinical trial. J Clin Med. 2020;9(8):2471.

Kubicek GJ, LaCouture T, Kaden M, Kim TW, Lerman N, Khrizman P, et al. Preoperative radiosurgery for soft tissue sarcoma. Am J Clin Oncol. 2018;41(1):86–9.

Leeman JE, Bilsky M, Laufer I, Folkert MR, Taunk NK, Osborne JR, et al. Stereotactic body radiotherapy for metastatic spinal sarcoma: a detailed patterns-of-failure study. J Neurosurg Spine. 2016;25(1):52–8.

Levine AM, Coleman C, Horasek S. Stereotactic radiosurgery for the treatment of primary sarcomas and sarcoma metastases of the spine. Neurosurgery. 2009;64(2 SUPPL):54–9.

Lindsay AD, Haupt EE, Chan CM, Spiguel AR, Scarborough MT, Zlotecki RA, et al. Treatment of sarcoma lung metastases with stereotactic body radiotherapy. Sarcoma. 2018;2018:10–5.

Marudanayagam R, Sandhu B, Perera MTPR, Bramhall SR, Mayer D, Buckels JAC, et al. Liver resection for metastatic soft tissue sarcoma: an analysis of prognostic factors. Eur J Surg Oncol. 2011;37(1):87–92. https://doi.org/10.1016/j.ejso.2010.11.006.

Mehta N, Selch M, Wang PC, Federman N, Lee JM, Eilber FC, et al. Safety and efficacy of stereotactic body radiation therapy in the treatment of pulmonary metastases from high grade sarcoma. Sarcoma. 2013;2013:360214.

Miller JA, Balagamwala EH, Angelov L, Suh JH, Djemil T, Magnelli A, et al. Stereotactic radiosurgery for the treatment of primary and metastatic spinal sarcomas. Technol Cancer Res Treat. 2017;16(3):276–84.

Naghavi AO, Fernandez DC, Mesko N, Juloori A, Martinez A, Scott JG, et al. American brachytherapy society consensus statement for soft tissue sarcoma brachytherapy. Brachytherapy. 2017;16(3):466–89. https://doi.org/10.1016/j.brachy.2017.02.004.

National Comprehensive Cancer Network. Soft tissue Sarcoma (Version 1.2021). 2021. https://www.nccn.org/professionals/physician_gls/pdf/sarcoma_blocks.pdf. Accessed 18 Mar 2021.

O'Sullivan B, Davis A, Turcotte R, Bell R, Catton C, Chabot P, et al. Preoperative versus postoperative radiotherapy in soft-tissue sarcoma of the limbs: a randomised trial. Lancet. 2002;359:2235–41.

Pawlik TM, Vauthey JN, Abdalla EK, Pollock RE, Ellis LM, Curley SA. Results of a single-center experience with resection and ablation for sarcoma metastatic to the liver. Arch Surg. 2006;141(6):537–43.

Pennington JD, Eilber FC, Eilber FR, Singh AS, Reed JP, Chmielowski B, et al. Long-term outcomes with Ifosfamide-based hypofractionated preoperative Chemoradiotherapy for extremity soft tissue sarcomas. Am J Clin Oncol. 2018;41(12):1154–61.

Petera J, Soumarová R, Růžičková J, Neumanová R, Dušek L, Sirák I, et al. Perioperative hyperfractionated high-dose rate brachytherapy for the treatment of soft tissue sarcomas: multicentric experience. Ann Surg Oncol. 2010;17(1):206–10.

Porter GA, Cantor SB, Walsh GL, Rusch VW, Leung DH, DeJesus AY, et al. Cost-effectiveness of pulmonary resection and systemic chemotherapy in the management of metastatic soft tissue sarcoma: a combined analysis from the University of Texas M. D. Anderson and Memorial Sloan-Kettering cancer centers. J Thorac Cardiovasc Surg. 2004;127(5):1366–72.

Savina M, Le Cesne A, Blay JY, Ray-Coquard I, Mir O, Toulmonde M, et al. Patterns of care and outcomes of patients with METAstatic soft tissue SARComa in a real-life setting: the METASARC observational study. BMC Med. 2017;15(1):1–11.

Sim AJ, Ahmed KA, Keller A, Figura NB, Oliver DE, Sarangkasiri S, et al. Outcomes and the role of primary histology following LINAC-based stereotactic radiation for sarcoma brain metastases. Am J Clin Oncol. 2020;43(5):356–61.

Soyfer V, Corn BW, Kollender Y, Issakov J, Dadia S, Flusser G, et al. Hypofractionated adjuvant radiation therapy of soft-tissue sarcoma achieves excellent results in elderly patients. Br J Radiol. 2013;86(1028):15–8.

Soyfer V, Corn BW, Shtraus N, Honig N, Meir Y, Kollender J, et al. Single-institution experience of SBRT for lung metastases in sarcoma patients. Am J Clin Oncol. 2017;40(1):83–5.

van Leeuwen CM, Oei AL, Crezee J, Bel A, Franken NAP, Stalpers LJA, et al. The alfa and beta of tumours: a review of parameters of the linear-quadratic model, derived from clinical radiotherapy studies. Radiat Oncol. 2018;13(96):1–11.

Wang D, Zhang Q, Eisenberg BL, Kane JM, Li XA, Lucas D, et al. Significant reduction of late toxicities in patients with extremity sarcoma treated with image-guided radiation therapy to a reduced target volume: results of radiation therapy oncology group RTOG-0630 trial. J Clin Oncol. 2015;33(20):2231–8.

Zagars GK, Ballo MT, Pisters PWT, Pollock RE, Patel SR, Benjamin RS, et al. Prognostic factors for patients with localized soft-tissue sarcoma treated with conservation surgery and radiation therapy: an analysis of 1225 patients. Cancer. 2003;97(10):2530–43.

Chapter 11
Extracranial Oligometastases

William C. Chen and Steve E. Braunstein

Pearls

- The term *oligometastasis* and concepts surrounding the idea of an *oligometastatic state* were most codified in a seminal editorial by Hellman and Weichselbaum in 1995, but substantial literature and debate predate this publication, dating back to 1969 or earlier (Hellman and Weichselbaum 1995; Rubin et al. 2006; Weichselbaum and Hellman 2011).
- The *oligometastatic state* describes a spectrum of metastatic disease states in which a small number of metastases (typical current definitions are five or fewer metastases) arise to clinical attention. Some undefined small proportion of these patients may be amenable to local metastasis-directed therapy (MDT) leading to long-term survival, which may constitute "cure." A greater proportion may also benefit from more durable disease control with MDT.

W. C. Chen · S. E. Braunstein (✉)
Department of Radiation Oncology, University of California, San Francisco, San Francisco, CA, USA
e-mail: william.chen@ucsf.edu; Steve.Braunstein@ucsf.edu

265

R. A. Sethi et al. (eds.), *Handbook of Evidence-Based Stereotactic Radiosurgery and Stereotactic Body Radiotherapy*, https://doi.org/10.1007/978-3-031-33156-5_11

- The spectrum of oligometastatic disease states is varied. One classification scheme proposed by Guckenberger and colleagues at the EORTC/ESTRO in 2020 divides cases by several characteristics: (Hellman and Weichselbaum 1995) *de novo* versus *repeat* versus *(treatment) induced* states, (Rubin et al. 2006) oligo*metastasis* versus *recurrence* versus *progression* versus *persistence*, and (Weichselbaum and Hellman 2011) *synchronous* versus *metachronous*. Oligometastatic class-specific outcomes are likely variable but are not yet well defined (Guckenberger et al. 2020).
- *Synchronous* disease is identified "simultaneously" with the primary tumor. For practical purposes, Guckenberger et al. defined a 6-month time window for identification of synchronous oligometastases. Oligometastases identified in the past 6 months would be defined as *metachronous* disease.
- Prior surgical series have reported 5-year survival rate of 25–50% after resection of lung or liver metastases, and 10–20-year survival rates of 15–25% in selected patients, suggesting that definitive treatment of oligometastases could contribute to long-term survival in a population selected for surgery (Tomlinson et al. 2007; Wei et al. 2006; Pastorino et al. 1997; Casiraghi et al. 2011; Abbas et al. 2011).
- Accumulating evidence suggests SBRT to be an effective option for extracranial MDT for a variety of locations (most commonly lung, liver, adrenal, bone, and lymph nodes) and may broaden the population of patients who are candidates for MDT. This paradigm is increasingly studied across a variety of primary tumor histologies, including prostate, colorectal, breast, NSCLC, melanoma, thyroid, renal/bladder, and sarcoma, among others.
- There is now emerging prospective, phase II evidence in support of the safety and efficacy of SBRT MDT for NSCLC, prostate, as well as mixed-histology settings

(Palma et al. 2020; Ost et al. 2020; Iyengar et al. 2018; Gomez et al. 2019; Phillips et al. 2020).

- It is increasingly clear that SBRT MDT can provide good local control, with modern dose-escalated studies reporting 2-year local control rates of 75–90% and 2- to 3-year disease-free survival (DFS) of 20–30% and rates of clinically significant (grade 3+) toxicity attributable to SBRT of 5% or less (Chalkidou et al. 2021; Lehrer et al. 2020), and prospective trials demonstrating improved progression-free survival (PFS) compared to usual care.
- While at least two phase II studies, SABR-COMET and Gomez et al., have also identified a possible overall survival benefit for SBRT MDT, phase III randomized studies are needed to confirm these findings (Palma et al. 2020; Gomez et al. 2019).

Treatment Indications

- Well-defined indications for SBRT MDT that apply universally across histologies and clinical settings are lacking, and recommendations for SBRT MDT should be individualized, ideally with multidisciplinary input.
- Factors that may contribute depending on the clinical scenario include age, performance status and comorbidity, "pace" of disease, disease burden (number of metastases, size/volume of metastases, number of organs involved, degree of organ impairment), degree of "systemic control" and response to systemic therapy, remaining systemic therapy options, patient goals of care, and predicted remaining life span.
- MDT SBRT may simultaneously achieve symptom palliation with similar efficacy and greater local control than palliative radiotherapy, but palliative radiotherapy may be better justified among patients with poor performance status and/or with limited prognosis (3 months or less).

- Select inclusion criteria used previously in prospective trials (criteria below are non-exhaustive; refer to primary protocols for full criteria) have been included:
  - **NSCLC**:
    - *Gomez* et al. and *NRG-LU002* (accruing): three or fewer synchronous oligometastases after stable disease or any response to frontline chemotherapy, ECOG 2 or lower, 18 years or older.
    - *UK SARON trial* (accruing): 18 years or older, ECOG 0–1, fully staged by PET-CT and MR/CT brain, three or fewer synchronous oligometastases, acceptable lung function and radiation plans which meet pre-specified constraints, and able to undergo cytotoxic chemotherapy (Conibear et al. 2018).
  - **Prostate**:
    - *STOMP*: three or fewer asymptomatic extracranial metachronous, hormone-sensitive or naïve metastases following biochemical recurrence after previous curative-intent radiation or surgery, WHO 0–1.
    - *ORIOLE*: three or fewer extracranial, metachronous, hormone-sensitive or naïve metastases following biochemical recurrence after previous curative-intent radiation or surgery, maximum size 5 cm and maximum volume 250 cc.
  - **Breast**:
    - *NRG-BR002* (accruing): four or fewer extracranial metastases diagnosed within 365 days of primary tumor, controlled primary, maximum metastasis size 5 cm and well demarcated, Zubrod 2 or lower.
  - **Mixed histology**:
    - *SABR-COMET*: five or fewer metastases (no more than three in one organ) with controlled primary tumor treated at least 3 months prior to the development of metastases, ECOG 0–1, life

expectancy at least 6 months, metastases amenable to SBRT.

- *UK registry study* (accruing): three or fewer metachronous extracranial metastases (at least 6 months from primary tumor), WHO 2 or lower, 18 years or older, life expectancy at least 6 months (Chalkidou et al. 2021).

Workup

- **H&P, Review of Systems, and Laboratories**:
  - These are performed every 3 months in patients with known metastatic disease. Please refer to site-specific chapters for details on site-specific evaluation.
- **Imaging**:
  - The role and frequency of interval systemic imaging (PET-CT or CTC/A/P ± contrast ± bone scan) to survey for development of metastatic disease in a symptomatic patient is not well defined. High-risk patients may benefit from surveillance imaging every 6 months for early detection of oligometastatic disease.
  - Patients diagnosed with metastatic disease should undergo systemic imaging (PET-CT or CTC/A/P ± contrast ± bone scan, brain MRI) to rule out additional lesions.
  - Refer to site-specific chapters for organ-specific imaging recommendations for radiation planning.
- **Pathology**.
  - The first site of metastasis or most accessible site is usually biopsied to confirm the metastatic state. Biopsies of additional lesions may be performed to confirm the sites of metastasis if involvement is unclear based on imaging, physical exam, and/or laboratory workup.

Radiosurgical Technique

- Please refer to site-specific chapters for simulation, planning, and dose delivery recommendations.

Toxicities and Management

- Please refer to site-specific chapters for organ system-specific toxicity profiles and management.

Recommended Follow-Up

- Repeat H&P and PET-CT or CTC/A/P + contrast and bone scan at least every 3 months starting 2–3 months after treatment to assess for response and progression of disease.

Evidence

Prospective Trials

- **NSCLC, Gomez trial, 2019**: Gomez et al. (2016, 2019): Multicenter, randomized, phase II trial, $N = 49$ NSCLC patients with three or fewer metastases with stable/partial response to frontline cytotoxic chemotherapy were randomized to local consolidative therapy (LCT), SBRT, and/or surgery, to all sites of disease followed by maintenance chemo vs. maintenance chemotherapy. Stopped early due to significant PFS benefit; with f/u of 38.8 months, PFS extended to 14.2 months with LCT vs. 4.4 months, and OS extended to 41.2 months vs. 9.4 months ($P = 0.034$). Only six patients had EGFR mutations (ongoing companion NORTHSTAR trial studying LCT for EGFR + NSCLC). No grade 4–5 toxicities occurred (Gomez et al. 2016, 2019).

- **NSCLC, UTSW trial, 2018**: Iyengar et al. (2018): Single-institution, randomized, phase II trial, $N = 29$ EGFR/ALK wild-type NSCLC patients with five or fewer stable/responding metastases after induction chemotherapy, randomized to SBRT to all sites plus chemo vs. maintenance chemotherapy alone. Trial stopped early due to significant PFS benefit with a median f/u of 9.6 months; PFS was 9.7 months with consolidative SBRT vs. 3.5 months ($P = 0.01$). Toxicity was equivalent, with $N = 4$ grade 3 toxicities on the SBRT arm, and no treatment-related deaths (Iyengar et al. 2018).

- **Mixed histology, SABR-COMET, phase II**: Palma et al. (2019, 2020): Multicenter, randomized, phase II trial, $N = 99$ patients (mixed histology) with five or fewer metastases, life expectancy of at least 6 months, and controlled primary tumor (see inclusion criteria above) were randomized 2:1 to MDT SBRT vs. usual care. With a median f/u of 51 months, MDT resulted in increased OS, with 5-year OS of 42.3% vs. 17.7% ($P = 0.006$). A trend towards OS benefit remained after examining non-prostate cancer patients only (33.1% vs. 16.2%, $P = 0.085$). Notably, overall local control was 63% in the SBRT arm, with relatively low rates of local control for lung (51%) and liver (50%) metastases. 4.5% of SBRT patients died from treatment, two from pulmonary complications and one from surgical complication related to a gastric ulcer. One main criticism of this trial is the imbalance in the number of prostate cancer patients among arms, favoring the SBRT arm (Palma et al. 2019, 2020).

- **Mixed histology, UK prospective observational trial**: Chalkidou et al. (2021): Multicenter, national registry, single-arm prospective observational trial, run in the UK, $N = 1422$ patients with one to three extracranial metachronous metastases identified at least 6 months from primary tumor treatment, life expectancy of at least 6 months, and ECOG 2 or lower were treated with SBRT (24–60 Gy in 3–8 fractions). Prostate (28.6%), colorectal (27.9%), renal cell (10.1%), breast (5.5%), and lung (4.5%) histologies were included. Most common sites treated were nodes (31.3%), lung (29.3%), bone (12%), and liver (9.6%). 75.6% of patients had a single metastasis. Remarkably, 1-year OS was 92.3%, and 2-year OS was 79.2%, with a median f/u of 13 months. One-year OS was 80.2% for lung cancer and 93.7% for breast cancer. $N = 11$ (0.8%) grade 4 toxicities (most commonly ALT/bilirubin increases), and $N = 74$ (5.2%) grade 3 toxicities occurred, most commonly fatigue ($N = 28$). Excluding fatigue, the grade 3+ toxicity rate was 4.0%. No treatment-related deaths were observed (Chalkidou et al. 2021).

- **Prostate, ORIOLE**: Phillips et al. (2020): Multicenter, randomized, phase II trial, $N = 54$ patients, one to three metastases by conventional staging (metachronous), no ADT within 6 months and <3 years total (see above for inclusion criteria), randomized to SBRT MDT vs. observation. PSMA PET was performed, but physicians were blinded. At 6 months, 19% of SBRT patients progressed (PSA/imaging/ADT initiation) vs. 61% of patients in the observation arm. If all PSMA-avid lesions were targeted, progression was lower (16% vs. 63%). No grade 3+ toxicity was identified (Phillips et al. 2020).
- **Prostate, STOMP:** Ost et al. (2020): Multicenter, randomized, phase II trial, $N = 62$ patients, ≤3 metachronous metastases by choline-PET, randomized to SBRT/ surgery to all sites of disease (met-directed therapy, MDT) vs. observation. SBRT dose was 30 Gy/3 fx. 54.8% of patients had nodal disease only, and 45.2% had non-nodal (almost all bone). At a median f/u of 5.3 years, 5-year ADT-free survival was 34% in the MDT arm vs. 8% ($P = 0.06$). Five-year castrate resistance freedom was 76% for MDT vs. 53% for observation ($P = 0.27$) (Ost et al. 2020).

- **Prostate, POPSTAR**: Siva et al. (2018): Single-institution, single-arm trial, $N = 33$ patients with 1–3 metachronous metastases by NaF PET-CT + conventional imaging were treated with 20 Gy × 1 (80% isodose line) SBRT to all sites of disease. 60.6% of men had bone-only disease. Two-year local control was 93%, while 2-year disease PFS was 39% and 2-year ADT freedom was 48%. Three percent ($N = 1$) of patients experienced grade 3 toxicity (Siva et al. 2018).

Meta-analyses

- **RCC metastases, SABR-ORCA**: Zaorsky ct al. (2019): $N = 1602$ patients in 28 studies of SBRT for both extracranial and intracranial RCC metastases. Median treatment volume was 59.7 cc for extracranial metastases and 2.3 cc for intracranial. One-year LC was 89 and 90% for extra/intracranial metastases. One-year OS was 86.8% for patients with extracranial metastases and 49.7% for those with intracranial metastases. Grade 3+ toxicity was 0.7% for extracranial and 1.1% for intracranial disease. Authors conclude that SBRT was highly efficacious and safe for metastasis-directed therapy in RCC. Single-fraction SBRT and higher dose were associated with greater LC (Zaorsky et al. 2019).
- **Adrenal metastases, mixed histology**: Chen et al. (2020): $N = 1006$ patients in 39 retrospective studies with a median f/u of 12 months. $N = 63$ patients with bilateral adrenal metastases were treated. Median BED-10 was 67 Gy, and median dose was 38 Gy in 5 fx. Pooled 1-year and 2-year LC rates were 82% and 63%, and 1-year and 2-year OS rates were 66% and 42%. A strong relationship between BED-10 and LC was found, and BED-10 of 100 Gy was predicted to correspond to 2-year LC of 85.6% based on meta-regression. Grade 3+ toxicity was 1.8% and was mostly bowel or

stomach ulcers and associated bleeds. Only five patients (0.5%) were reported to have developed grade 2 adrenal insufficiency, and one patient (0.1%) developed hypertensive crisis (Chen et al. 2020).

- *Surgery and IR ablation*: SBRT for adrenal metastases compares favorably to interventional radiology-based ablation, which is associated with a grade 3+ toxicity rate of 16.1%, and intraprocedural hypertensive crisis in 21.9% (Pan et al. 2020). Similarly, while surgical series have not reported detailed complication outcomes, the perioperative mortality was 3% in one series (Howell et al. 2013), and the rate of postoperative adrenal insufficiency was 27% in another series (Heinrich et al. 2019), many of whom had severe insufficiency requiring prolonged hydrocortisone replacement.
- **Mixed sites, histologies**: Lehrer et al. (2020): $N = 943$ patients treated on 21 prospective trials with mixed primary histologies, with ≤5 metastases treated with SBRT (at least 5 Gy per fraction and eight or fewer fractions). Histologies were most commonly prostate (22.9%), colorectal (16.6%), breast (13.1%), and lung (12.8%). Acute grade 3+ toxicity was 1.2%, and late grade 3+ toxicity was 1.7%. Remarkably, the rate of pooled 1-year LC was 94.7% and 1-year OS was 85.4% (Lehrer et al. 2020).

References

Abbas S, Lam V, Hollands M. Ten-year survival after liver resection for colorectal metastases: systematic review and meta-analysis. ISRN Oncol. 2011;2011:763245.

Casiraghi M, De Pas T, Maisonneuve P, Brambilla D, Ciprandi B, Galetta D, et al. A 10-year single-center experience on 708 lung metastasectomies: the evidence of the "international registry of lung metastases". J Thorac Oncol. 2011;6:1373.

Chalkidou A, Macmillan T, Grzeda MT, Peacock J, Summers J, Eddy S, et al. Stereotactic ablative body radiotherapy in patients with oligometastatic cancers: a prospective, registry-based, single-arm, observational, evaluation study. Lancet Oncol. 2021;22(1):98–106.

Chen WC, Baal JD, Baal U, Pai J, Gottschalk A, Boreta L, et al. Stereotactic body radiation therapy of adrenal metastases: a pooled meta-analysis and systematic review of 39 studies with 1006 patients. Int J Radiat Oncol Biol Phys. 2020;107:48.

Conibear J, Chia B, Ngai Y, Bates AT, Counsell N, Patel R, et al. Study protocol for the SARON trial: a multicentre, randomised controlled phase III trial comparing the addition of stereotactic ablative radiotherapy and radical radiotherapy with standard chemotherapy alone for oligometastatic non-small cell lung cancer. BMJ Open. 2018;8:e020690.

Gomez DR, Blumenschein GR, Lee JJ, Hernandez M, Ye R, Camidge DR, et al. Local consolidative therapy versus maintenance therapy or observation for patients with oligometastatic non-small-cell lung cancer without progression after first-line systemic therapy: a multicentre, randomised, controlled, phase 2 study. Lancet Oncol. 2016;17:1672.

Gomez DR, Tang C, Zhang J, Blumenschein GR, Hernandez M, Jack Lee J, et al. Local consolidative therapy vs. maintenance therapy or observation for patients with oligometastatic non-small-cell lung cancer: long-term results of a multi-institutional, phase II, randomized study. J Clin Oncol. 2019;37:1558.

Guckenberger M, Lievens Y, Bouma AB, Collette L, Dekker A, deSouza NM, et al. Characterisation and classification of oligometastatic disease: a European Society for Radiotherapy and Oncology and European Organisation for Research and Treatment of Cancer consensus recommendation. Lancet Oncol. 2020;21:e18.

Heinrich DA, Adolf C, Holler F, Lechner B, Schneider H, Riester A, et al. Adrenal insufficiency after unilateral adrenalectomy in primary Aldosteronism: long-term outcome and clinical impact. J Clin Endocrinol Metab. 2019;104:5658.

Hellman S, Weichselbaum RR. Oligometastases. J Clin Oncol. 1995;13(1):8–10.

Howell GM, Carty SE, Armstrong MJ, Stang MT, McCoy KL, Bartlett DL, et al. Outcome and prognostic factors after adrenalectomy for patients with distant adrenal metastasis. Ann Surg Oncol. 2013;20:3491.

Iyengar P, Wardak Z, Gerber DE, Tumati V, Ahn C, Hughes RS, et al. Consolidative radiotherapy for limited metastatic non-small-cell lung cancer: a phase 2 randomized clinical trial. JAMA Oncol. 2018;4:e173501.

Lehrer EJ, Singh R, Wang M, Chinchilli VM, Trifiletti DM, Ost P, et al. Safety and survival rates associated with ablative stereotactic radiotherapy for patients with oligometastatic cancer. JAMA Oncol. 2020;7:92.

Ost P, Reynders D, Decaestecker K, Fonteyne V, Lumen N, De Bruycker A, et al. Surveillance or metastasis-directed therapy for oligometastatic prostate cancer recurrence (STOMP): five-year results of a randomized phase II trial. J Clin Oncol. 2020;38:10.

Palma DA, Olson R, Harrow S, Gaede S, Louie AV, Haasbeek C, et al. Stereotactic ablative radiotherapy versus standard of care palliative treatment in patients with oligometastatic cancers (SABR-COMET): a randomised, phase 2, open-label trial. Lancet. 2019;393:2051.

Palma DA, Olson R, Harrow S, Gaede S, Louie AV, Haasbeek C, et al. Stereotactic ablative radiotherapy for the comprehensive treatment of oligometastatic cancers: long-term results of the SABR-COMET phase II randomized trial. J Clin Oncol. 2020;38:2830.

Pan S, Baal JD, Chen WC, Baal U, Pai J, Baal J, et al. Image-guided percutaneous ablation of adrenal metastases: a systematic review and meta-analysis. J Vasc Interv Radiol. 2020;32:527.

Pastorino U, Buyse M, Friedel G, Ginsberg RJ, Girard P, Goldstraw P, et al. Long-term results of lung metastasectomy: prognostic analyses based on 5206 cases. J Thorac Cardiovasc Surg. 1997;113:37.

Phillips R, Shi WY, Deek M, Radwan N, Lim SJ, Antonarakis ES, et al. Outcomes of observation vs stereotactic ablative radiation for oligometastatic prostate cancer: the ORIOLE phase 2 randomized clinical trial. JAMA Oncol. 2020;6:650.

Rubin P, Brasacchio R, Katz A. Solitary metastases: illusion versus reality. Semin Radiat Oncol. 2006;16(2):120–30.

Siva S, Bressel M, Murphy DG, Shaw M, Chander S, Violet J, et al. Stereotactic ablative body radiotherapy (SABR) for Oligometastatic prostate cancer: a prospective clinical trial. Eur Urol. 2018;74:455.

Tomlinson JS, Jarnagin WR, DeMatteo RP, Fong Y, Kornprat P, Gonen M, et al. Actual 10-year survival after resection of colorectal liver metastases defines cure. J Clin Oncol. 2007;25:4575.

Wei AC, Greig PD, Grant D, Taylor B, Langer B, Gallinger S. Survival after hepatic resection for colorectal metastases: a 10-year experience. Ann Surg Oncol. 2006;13:668.

Weichselbaum RR, Hellman S. Oligometastases revisited. Nat Rev Clin Oncol. 2011;8:378.

Zaorsky NG, Lehrer EJ, Kothari G, Louie AV, Siva S. Stereotactic ablative radiation therapy for oligometastatic renal cell carcinoma (SABR ORCA): a meta-analysis of 28 studies. Eur Urol Oncol. 2019;2:515.

Appendix A: Dose-Volume Criteria

Igor Barani

Tissue	Maximum critical volume in excess of threshold	One fraction		Three fractions		Five fractions		Endpoint (≥grade 3)
		Threshold dose (Gy)	Maximum point dose (Gy)	Threshold dose (Gy)	Maximum point dose (Gy)	Threshold dose (Gy)	Maximum point dose (Gy)	
Optic pathway	<0.2 cc	8	12	15.3 (5.1 Gy/fx)	17.4 (5.8 Gy/fx)	23 (4.6 Gy/fx)	25 (5 Gy/fx)	Neuritis
Cochlea	–	–	9	–	17.1 (5.7 Gy/fx)	–	25 (5 Gy/fx)	Hearing loss
Brain stem (not medulla)	<0.5 cc	15	18	18 (6 Gy/fx)	23.1 (7.7 Gy/fx)	23 (4.6 Gy/fx)	31 (6.2 Gy/fx)	Cranial neuropathy
Spinal cord + medulla	<0.1 cc	10	14	18 (6 Gy/fx)	21 (7 Gy/fx)	23 (4.6 Gy/fx)	30 (6 Gy/fx)	Myelitis
Cauda equina	<5 cc	14	16	21.9 (7.3 Gy/fx)	24 (8 Gy/fx)	30 (6 Gy/fx)	32 (6.4 Gy/fx)	Neuritis
Sacral plexus	<5 cc	14.4	16	22.5 (7.5 Gy/fx)	24 (8 Gy/fx)	30 (6 Gy/fx)	32 (6.4 Gy/fx)	Neuropathy

| Tissue | Maximum critical volume in excess of threshold | One fraction | | Three fractions | | Five fractions | | Endpoint (≥grade 3) |
		Threshold dose (Gy)	Maximum point dose (Gy)	Threshold dose (Gy)	Maximum point dose (Gy)	Threshold dose (Gy)	Maximum point dose (Gy)	
Brachial plexus	<3 cc	–	24	–	27 (9 Gy/fx)	27 (5.4 Gy/fx)	30.5 (6.1 Gy/fx)	Neuropathy
Lung (right and left)	1500 cc	7	–	11.6 (3.87 Gy/fx)	–	12.5 Gy (2.5 Gy/fx)	–	Basic lung function
Lung (right and left)	1000 cc	7.4	–	12.4 (4.13 Gy/fx)	–	13.5 Gy (2.7 Gy/fx)	–	Pneumonitis
Bronchi, large (including trachea)	<4 cc	10.5	20.2	15 (5 Gy/fx)	30 (10 Gy/fx)	16.5 (3.3 Gy/fx)	40 (8 Gy/fx)	Stenosis/fistula
Bronchi, small	<0.5 cc	12.4	13.3	18.9 (6.3 Gy/fx)	23.1 (7.7 Gy/fx)	21 (4.2 Gy/fx)	33 (6.6 Gy/fx)	Stenosis w/ atelectasis
Chest wall	<1 cc	22	30	28.8 (9.6 Gy/fx)	36.9 (12.3 Gy/fx)	35 (7 Gy/fx)	43 (8.6 Gy/fx)	Pain or fracture

Tissue	Maximum critical volume in excess of threshold	One fraction Threshold dose (Gy)	One fraction Maximum point dose (Gy)	Three fractions Threshold dose (Gy)	Three fractions Maximum point dose (Gy)	Five fractions Threshold dose (Gy)	Five fractions Maximum point dose (Gy)	Endpoint (≥grade 3)
Chest wall	<30 cc	–	–	30 (10 Gy/fx)	–	–	–	Pain or fracture
Chest wall	<10 cc	–	–	30 (10 Gy/fx) (Rusthoven et al. 2009)	–	–	–	Pain or fracture
Chest wall	<71 cc to 2 cm chest wall contour	–	–	30 (10 Gy/fx)	–	30 (6 Gy/fx)	–	Pain or fracture
Esophagus	<5 cc	11.9	15.4	17.7 (5.9 Gy/fx)	25.2 (8.4 Gy/fx)	19.5 (3.9 Gy/fx)	35 (7 Gy/fx)	Stenosis/fistula
Stomach	<10 cc	11.2	12.4	16.5 (5.5 Gy/fx)	22.2 (7.4 Gy/fx)	18 (3.6 Gy/fx)	32 (6.4 Gy/fx)	Ulceration/fistula

Tissue	Maximum critical volume in excess of threshold	One fraction		Three fractions		Five fractions		Endpoint (≧grade 3)
		Threshold dose (Gy)	Maximum point dose (Gy)	Threshold dose (Gy)	Maximum point dose (Gy)	Threshold dose (Gy)	Maximum point dose (Gy)	
Stomach	<4%	22.5 (Chang et al. 2009)	–	–	30 (10 Gy/fx) (Kavanagh et al. 2010)	–	–	Ulceration
Stomach/bowel	Circumference	–	12	–	–	–	–	Ulceration/fistula
Small bowel	<30 cc	12.5 (Kavanagh et al. 2010)	–	–	30 (10 Gy/fx) (Kavanagh et al. 2010)	–	–	Ulceration/fistula
Duodenum	<5 cc	11.2	12.4	16.5 (5.5 Gy/fx)	22.2 (7.4 Gy/fx)	18 (3.6 Gy/fx)	32 (6.4 Gy/fx)	Ulceration
Duodenum	<10 cc	9	–	11.4 (3.8 Gy/fx)	–	12.5 Gy (2.5 Gy/fx)	–	Ulceration
Duodenum	<5%	22.5 (Chang et al. 2009)	–	–	–	–	–	Ulceration

Tissue	Maximum critical volume in excess of threshold	One fraction Threshold dose (Gy)	One fraction Maximum point dose (Gy)	Three fractions Threshold dose (Gy)	Three fractions Maximum point dose (Gy)	Five fractions Threshold dose (Gy)	Five fractions Maximum point dose (Gy)	Endpoint (≥grade 3)
Jejunum/ileum	<5 cc	11.9	15.4	17.7 (5.9 Gy/fx)	25.2 (8.4 Gy/fx)	19.5 (3.9 Gy/fx)	35 (7 Gy/fx)	Enteritis/obstruction
Colon	<20 cc	14.3	18.4	24 (8 Gy/fx)	28.2 (9.4 Gy/fx)	25 (5 Gy/fx)	38 (7.6 Gy/fx)	Colitis/fistula
Rectum	<20 cc	14.3	16	24 (8 Gy/fx)	28.2 (9.4 Gy/fx)	25 (5 Gy/fx)	38 (7.6 Gy/fx)	Proctitis/fistula
Rectum	Circumference	–	14	–	–	–	–	Proctitis/fistula
Rectum	<1 cc	–	–	–	–	36 (12 Gy/fx) (McBride et al. 2012)	–	Proctitis/fistula
Bladder	<15 cc	11.4	18.4	16.8 (5.6 Gy/fx)	28.2 (9.4 Gy/fx)	18.3 (3.65 Gy/fx)	38 (7.6 Gy/fx)	Cystitis/fistula

Tissue	Maximum critical volume in excess of threshold	One fraction		Three fractions		Five fractions		Endpoint (≧grade 3)
		Threshold dose (Gy)	Maximum point dose (Gy)	Threshold dose (Gy)	Maximum point dose (Gy)	Threshold dose (Gy)	Maximum point dose (Gy)	
Bladder	–	–	–	–	–	–	54	Cystitis/fistula
Penile bulb	<3 cc	14	34	21.9 (7.3 Gy/fx)	42 (14 Gy/fx)	30 (6 Gy/fx)	50 (10 Gy/fx)	Impotence
Urethra	<10%	–	–	–	–	49 (9.8 Gy/fx) (McBride et al. 2012)	55	Urethral stricture
Femoral heads (right and left)	<10 cc	14	–	21.9 (7.3 Gy/fx)	–	30 (6 Gy/fx)	41.8 (8.36 Gy/fx)	Necrosis
Femoral head	<5 cc	–	–	–	–	25 (5 Gy/fx)	–	Necrosis
Kidney	<2/3 Volume	10.6	–	18.6 (6.2 Gy/fx)	–	23 (4.6 Gy/fx)	–	Malignant hypertension

Tissue	Maximum critical volume in excess of threshold	One fraction Threshold dose (Gy)	One fraction Maximum point dose (Gy)	Three fractions Threshold dose (Gy)	Three fractions Maximum point dose (Gy)	Five fractions Threshold dose (Gy)	Five fractions Maximum point dose (Gy)	Endpoint ($\geqq$grade 3)
Kidney (must meet *both* constraints)	<33% of *spared* kidney volume	10	–	15 (5 Gy/fx)	–	18 (3.6 Gy/ fx)	–	Malignant hypertension
	<35% of *total* kidney volume	10	–	15 (5 Gy/fx)	–	18 (3.6 Gy/ fx)	–	
Kidney	<75% of closest kidney volume	5 (Goodman et al. 2010)	–	–	–	–	–	Not specified
Liver	<700 cc	9.1	–	19.2 (6.4 Gy/ fx)	–	21 (4.2 Gy/ fx)	–	Basic liver function

Tissue	Maximum critical volume in excess of threshold	One fraction			Three fractions			Five fractions		Endpoint (≧grade 3)
		Threshold dose (Gy)	Maximum point dose (Gy)		Threshold dose (Gy)	Maximum point dose (Gy)		Threshold dose (Gy)	Maximum point dose (Gy)	
Liver	<70%	–	–		–	–		30 (6 Gy/fx) (Katz et al. 2007)	–	Cirrhosis/hepatitis
Liver	<50%	5 (Chang et al. 2009)	–		–	–		–	–	Biliary stricture
	<75%	2.5 (Chang et al. 2009)								
Liver	Mean	–	–		HCC:13 (4.3 Gy/fx) (Pan et al. 2010) Metastasis: 18 (6 Gy/fx) (Pan et al. 2010)	–		–	–	Radiation-induced liver disease (RILD)

Tissue	Maximum critical volume in excess of threshold	One fraction		Three fractions		Five fractions		Endpoint (≧grade 3)
		Threshold dose (Gy)	Maximum point dose (Gy)	Threshold dose (Gy)	Maximum point dose (Gy)	Threshold dose (Gy)	Maximum point dose (Gy)	
Heart	<15 cc	16	22	24 (8 Gy/fx)	30 (10 Gy/fx)	32 (6.4 Gy/fx)	38 (7.6 Gy/fx)	Pericarditis
Great vessels	<10 cc	31	37	39 (13 Gy/fx)	45 (15 Gy/fx)	47 |(9.4 Gy/fx)	53 (10.6 Gy/fx)	Aneurysm

Source: This table summarizes tolerance doses that are largely based on the AAPM Task Group Report 101 (AAPM TG 101) as well as other sources of primary data, including our own institutional experience (Timmerman 2008a, b; Dunlap et al. 2010; Wersäll et al. 2005; Benedict et al. 2010; Timmerman et al. 2007; Chang and Timmerman 2007; Murphy et al. 2010). Other sources of primary information are cited specifically if based on smaller reports or early data from limited experience. Please note that most of the doses are unvalidated and based either on toxicity observations or on mathematical models, and there is a good measure of subjectivity involved as well. Because of the relative absence of long-term follow-up data for SBRT, it should be recognized that the tolerance data in the table is merely an approximation of normal tissue tolerance. When treating in areas where there is sparse or absent literature support for toxicity and complications, it is strongly recommended that formal institutional guidelines and prospective clinical trials with close oversight are implemented

References

Benedict SH, Yenice KM, Followill D, Galvin JM, Hinson W, et al. Stereotactic body radiation therapy: the report of AAPM Task Group 101. Med Phys. 2010;37:4078–101.

Chang BK, Timmerman RD. Stereotactic body radiation therapy: a comprehensive review. Am J Clin Oncol. 2007;30:637–44.

Chang DT, Schellenberg D, Shen J, Kim J, Goodman KA, et al. Stereotactic radiotherapy for unresectable adenocarcinoma of the pancreas. Cancer. 2009;115:665–72.

Dunlap NE, Cai J, Biedermann GB, Yang W, Benedict SH, et al. Chest wall volume receiving >30 Gy predicts risk of severe pain and/or rib fracture after lung stereotactic body radiotherapy. Int J Radiat Oncol Biol Phys. 2010;76:796–801.

Goodman KA, Wiegner EA, Maturen KE, Zhang Z, Mo Q, et al. Dose-escalation study of single-fraction stereotactic body radiotherapy for liver malignancies. Int J Radiat Oncol Biol Phys. 2010;78:486–93.

Katz AW, Carey-Sampson M, Muhs AG, Milano MT, Schell MC, Okunieff P. Hypofractionated stereotactic body radiation therapy (SBRT) for limited hepatic metastases. Int J Radiat Oncol Biol Phys. 2007;67:793–8.

Kavanagh BD, Pan CC, Dawson LA, Das SK, Li XA, et al. Radiation dose-volume effects in the stomach and small bowel. Int J Radiat Oncol Biol Phys. 2010;76:S101–7.

McBride SM, Wong DS, Dombrowski JJ, Harkins B, Tapella P, et al. Hypofractionated stereotactic body radiotherapy in low-risk prostate adenocarcinoma: preliminary results of a multi-institutional phase 1 feasibility trial. Cancer. 2012;118:3681–90.

Murphy JD, Christman-Skieller C, Kim J, Dieterich S, Chang DT, Koong AC. A dosimetric model of duodenal toxicity after stereotactic body radiotherapy for pancreatic cancer. Int J Radiat Oncol Biol Phys. 2010;78:1420–6.

Pan CC, Kavanagh BD, Dawson LA, Li XA, Das SK, et al. Radiation-associated liver injury. Int J Radiat Oncol Biol Phys. 2010;76:S94–100.

Rusthoven KE, Kavanagh BD, Burri SH, Chen C, Cardenes H, et al. Multi-institutional phase I/II trial of stereotactic body radiation therapy for lung metastases. J Clin Oncol. 2009;27:1579–84.

Timmerman RD. An overview of hypofractionation and introduction to this issue of seminars in radiation oncology. Semin Radiat Oncol. 2008a;18:215–22.

Timmerman RD. An overview of hypofractionation and introduction to this issue of seminars in radiation oncology. Semin Radiat Oncol. 2008b;18:215–22.

Timmerman RD, Kavanagh BD, Cho LC, Papiez L, Xing L. Stereotactic body radiation therapy in multiple organ sites. J Clin Oncol. 2007;25:947–52.

Wersäll PJ, Blomgren H, Lax I, Kälkner KM, Linder C, et al. Extracranial stereotactic radiotherapy for primary and metastatic renal cell carcinoma. Radiother Oncol. 2005;77:88–95.

Index

A

Abdominal compression, 141, 154
Acoustic neuroma, 4, 6, 41, 50, 55, 68
Acromegaly, 49, 70
ACTH, 42, 48
Active breathing control (ABC), 154
Acute toxicities, 62, 183, 184
Adaptive RT (ART) planning, 16
Adenocarcinoma, 138
Adrenal metastases, 138
Alcohol, 122
Alkaline phosphatase, 122, 138
Alopecia, 54
American Medical Association (AMA), 7
Amygdala, 79
Analgesics, 126, 146
Anaplastic meningioma, 40, 65
Aneurysm, 44, 128
Angiogram, 55
Anterior fossa, 63
Antimicrobial, 126
Arteriovenous malformation (AVM), 43–44, 48, 49, 53, 55, 72–74
Ataxia, 42
Audiometry, 55

B

Beam energy, 15
Beam geometry, 16
Beam shaping, 15
Bcam stability test, 29
Biologically effective dose (BED), 164
Biopsy, 41
Bitemporal hemianopsia, 42
Bleeding, 54, 74
Blocking, 76
Blood-brain barrier, 48
Bone, 41, 269, 270
Borderline resectable disease (BRPC), 162
Brachial plexopathy, 126, 146
Brachial plexus, 126, 138, 146
Brachytherapy (BT), 127
    dose delivery, 237
    dose limitations, 236
    dose prescription, 236
    follow-up, 238
    recommended imaging, 235
    simulation and treatment planning, 235–236
    toxicities and management, 237–238
    treatment indications, 234–235

work-up, 235
Bragg-peak protons, 3
Brain metastasis, 4, 40, 57, 259
Brain necrosis, 54, 127
Brainstem, 51, 77
Breast cancers, 2, 5, 40
Bromocriptine, 47
Bronchiectasis, 155
Bronchodilator, 146
Bronchoscopic biopsy, 139

C
Cabergoline, 47
Calvarium, 68
Cardiopulmonary dysfunction, 145
Carotid, 61, 128, 132
Carotid artery stenosis, 61
Cavernous malformations, 43, 54, 75
Cavernous sinus, 42
Centers for Medicare and Medicaid Services (CMS), 7
Cerebellopontine angle (CPA), 41, 44, 55, 66
Cerebral aneurysm, 43
Cerebral vasculopathy, 70
Cetuximab, 131, 132
Chemodectomas, 42
Chemoradiation, 130, 139
Chemoreceptors, 42
Chemotherapy, 131
Chest pain, 145
Chest wall, 139, 141
Choline, 48
Chordoma, 93, 106–108
Choriocarcinoma, 48
Chromosome 22q, 41
Cisplatin, 128
Clinically localized prostate cancer
    checklist, 209–210
    contouring, 212–215
    evidence, 216–220

follow-up, 216
image guidance, 212–215
indications and work-up, 210–211
simulation, 211–212
treatment planning, 212–215
Clival chordoma SBRT, 96
CN, 41, 44, 61, 65, 67, 68, 70
CNS, 45
Common acute toxicities, 143
Comorbidities, 145
Complications, 61, 70, 73
Concurrent systemic therapy, 131–133, 184
Conformality index, 59
Conjunctival injection, 44
Contrast, 49, 269
Control rate, 63, 67, 70
Conventional EBRT, 101–102
Cough, 138, 145, 146
Cranial nerve, 54
Cranial nerve palsies, 42
Craniofacial pain syndrome, 45
Craniopharyngiomas, 45
Critical structures, 50, 62
CSF leak, 70
CSS, 61, 62
CT-guided biopsy, 138
CTV, 141
Cumulative dose, 78, 127
Current Procedural Terminology, 7
Cushing disease, 70
Cyberknife robotic radiosurgery, 29
CyberKnife system, 29
Cyclotron, 2
Cyst, 62, 71

D
Death, 42, 75, 79
Demyelination, 44, 49
Dermatitis, 126, 145
Digestive system
    dose prescription, 175–178

evidence, 186–196
HCC, 166
ICC, 167
liver-directed locoregional
    therapies, 167–170
liver SBRT, 164–165
pancreatic cancer, 165–166
pancreatic SBRT, 163–164
recommended follow-up, 185
simulation and field design,
    171–174
target delineation, 172
toxicities and management,
    183–185
treatment delivery, 178–183
treatment options for, 167
Dmax, 144
Dose, 50–53, 56, 124, 125, 143
conformity, 15
constraints, 179–182
escalation, 53, 189
gradient, 15
heterogeneity, 15
prescription, 124
reduction, 51
Dosimetric quality assurance, 26
Dural tail sign, 49
Dysesthesias, 77
Dysphagia, 80, 122, 126, 132
Dyspnea, 138, 145, 146

E
ECOG performance status, 58
Edema, 48, 54, 63
EGFR mutation, 139
Eloquent, 43, 72, 73
EORTC, 57
Epilepsy, 45, 79
Esophageal stricture, 126, 146
Esophagitis, 145
Esophagus, 142
Essential tremor, 45, 80
External beam radiation therapy
    (EBRT), 123
Extracranial oligometastases

follow-up, 270
indications, 267–269
prospective trials, 270–274
radiosurgical technique, 270
toxicities and management,
    270
work-up, 269
Eye dryness, 54

F
Facial nerve, 42
Facial numbness, 44, 69, 76, 128
Facial palsy, 54
Facial paresis, 42
Facial paresthesia, 76
Fatigue, 54, 125, 143, 145
Fever, 145
Fibrosis, 132, 147, 155
Fiducial, 68
Fistula, 132, 146
Fletcher, Gilbert, 5
Fluid attenuation inversion
    recovery (FLAIR), 48
Foramen magnum, 49
Forbes-Albright syndrome, 42
Forward planning, 16
Fractionated, 62, 64, 68, 70
Fractionated conformal
    radiotherapy (FCRT),
    104
Free-breathing, 141
Free cortisol, 48
Functional adenoma, 71
Functional status, 62
Fusion, 49

G
Gadolinium, 48, 49
Gamma knife, 2
Gamma knife radiosurgery
    (GKRS), 44, 56–58, 62,
    63, 65–67, 69, 70, 72, 74,
    76–80
Gaze palsy, 79

Germ cell tumors, 79
Glial tumors, 45
Gliosis, 48
Glomus tumors, 42
Gross tumor volume (GTV), 50

H
Handwriting score, 80
Headache, 44
Head and neck cancer
    concurrent systemic therapy,
        131–133
    dose delivery, 125
    dose limitations, 124–125
    dose prescription, 124
    elderly/medically unfit, 133
    follow-up, 127
    laryngeal carcinoma, 129–130
    nasopharyngeal carcinoma,
        127–128
    oropharyngeal carcinoma,
        128–129
    postoperative, 129
    simulation and treatment
        planning, 123–124
    toxicities and management,
        125–127
    treatment indications, 123
Head and neck squamous cell
        carcinoma (HNSCC),
        121, 130
Hearing loss, 41, 69
Hearing preservation, 52, 67, 68
Heart, 142
Hemoptysis, 126, 138, 147
Hemorrhage, 72, 73, 75, 126, 127,
        132, 147
Hepatocellular carcinoma
        (HCC), 162, 166
Heterogeneity, 124, 131
Hippocampus, 79
Histology, 55, 61
Hoarseness, 138
Hopkins Verbal Learning Test, 57

Hormone, 43, 70, 71
Hormone replacement therapy,
        71
HPV, 122
Hydrocephalus, 42
Hyperbaric oxygen, 126, 146
Hyperesthesia, 54, 76
Hyperostosis, 49
Hypofractionation, 45, 69–71
Hypopharynx, 130
Hypopituitarism, 70, 71
Hypoxia, 145

I
iGTV, 141
Image-guided radiation therapy
        (IGRT) imaging
        systems, 22–25
Imaging, 54, 55, 269
Imaging-based treatment
        planning, 1
Immobilization, 4, 50
Impotence, 42
Initial definitive radiotherapy,
        241–243
Intensity modulated
        radiation therapy
        (IMRT), 1, 16
Intracranial tumor, 40–42, 50
Intrahepatic cholangiocarcinoma
        (ICC), 162, 167
Inverse planning, 16
Isocenter, 50, 77
Isodose line, 53, 68
Isointense, 49
ITV, 141

J
JROSG, 56

K
KPS, 40, 45, 46, 55–57

L

Lactate, 48
Landmark-based registration
    algorithm, 77
Laryngeal carcinoma, 129–130
Larynx, 130
Latency period, 72, 73
Leptomeningeal, 79
Lidocaine, 126, 145
Lifetime risk of hemorrhage, 43
Linear accelerator, 3, 56, 73
Liver-directed locoregional
    therapies, 167–170
Liver metastasis, 177–178, 184,
    185, 259, 266
Liver SBRT, 164–165, 171, 174,
    178–185, 191–196
Long-term toxicities, 183, 184
Lung, 142, 144
Lung cancer, 5, 40, 146
Lung metastases, 256–257
Lung SBRT
    dose delivery, 143
    dose limitations, 143
    dose prescription, 142–143,
        152
    evidence, 148–152
    follow-up, 147, 154–155
    motion management, 153–154
    simulation and treatment
        planning, 141–142
    toxicities and management,
        143–147
    treatment indications,
        139–141
    treatment planning, 152–153

M

Magnetic resonance imaging
    (MRI), 44, 48–50, 54,
    55, 79, 126, 269
Magnetic resonance
    spectroscopy, 48
Malnutrition, 132

Maximum Intensity Projection
    (MIP), 141
Maximum tolerated dose, 56
Mediastinoscopy, 139
Medulloblastoma, 45
Meiosis, 44
Melanoma, 40, 48
Memory impairment, 54
Meninges, 49
Meningioma, 41, 44, 48, 55, 62, 64,
    66
Metastasis, 40, 269
Metastatic STS, 255–259
Microadenoma, 42
Microvascular decompression, 47,
    76
MMSE, 57
Monte Carlo, 142
Movement disorders, 2, 4
MRA, 49
MRI-guided RT, 191
MRI-guided systems, 30
MTD, 56
Mucositis, 126, 132
Multivariate analysis, 55, 56, 59,
    62, 73, 76

N

N-acetylaspartic acid (NAA), 48
Nasal congestion, 44
Nasopharyngeal carcinoma,
    127–128
Nasopharynx, 130
Necrosis, 3, 48, 49, 54, 126–128
Nelson syndrome, 70
Neuralgia, 50, 53, 76
Neurectomy, 76
Neurocognitive testing, 57
Neuroendocrine tumor, 42
Neuropathic pain, 126, 146
Neurotoxicity, 56
Non-functioning pituitary
    adenomas, 71
Noninvasive immobilization, 97

North American Gamma Knife
  Consortium (NAGKC),
  65

O

Obliteration, 43, 53, 72–74
Obstruction, 42
Occupational therapy, 126, 146
Oligometastases, 238–241, 265
Oligometastasis-directed therapy,
  220–221
Oligometastatic state, 265
Optic chiasm, 42
Oral cavity, 130
Oropharyngeal carcinoma,
  128–129
Oropharynx, 130
Orthotopic liver transplantation
  (OLT), 162
Osteoradionecrosis, 127

P

Pain, 42, 44, 45, 47–49, 55, 76–78,
  126
Pain syndromes, 2, 4, 48
Pancoast, 138
Pancreatic cancer, 165–166, 175,
  185
Pancreatic SBRT, 163–164, 171,
  172, 178, 196
Papillary epithelial tumors, 79
Paraganglioma, 42, 52, 69
Parahippocampal gyrus, 79
Paranasal sinus, 130
Parkinson disease, 45, 80
Percent depth dose (PDD), 28
Performance status, 58, 122
Peri-orbital edema, 54
Peritumoral edema, 66
PET, 269
Petroclival meningioma, 66
Pharmacotherapy, 126, 145,
  146
Photon beam systems, 28

Pineal parenchymal tumors, 45,
  78, 79
Pineal tumor, 53
Pineoblastoma, 78
Pineocytoma, 78
Pituitary adenoma, 47–49, 52, 55
Pituitary infundibulum, 42
Pleural effusion, 138, 139
Pneumonitis, 145, 146
Pons, 50
Post-obstructive pneumonia, 138
Primary spine tumor, 95
Primary STS, 252–254
Primary tumors, 106–108
Prolactin, 42, 48
Prolactinoma, 42, 70
Prolactin-secreting, 47
Prostate cancer, 5, 220–221
Proton, 68
Pterygopalatine ganglion, 44, 45
Ptosis, 44
PTV, 141
Pulmonary function testing, 139
Pulmonary oligometastases, 140

R

Radiation-induced liver injury
  (RILD), 184
Radiation-induced myelopathy,
  112
Radiation therapy (RT), 161
Radiation Therapy Oncology
  Group (RTOG), 40, 55,
  56, 64, 141
Radiofrequency ablation (RFA),
  77, 163
Radionecrosis, 3, 56, 79
Radiosurgery, 2, 4, 48–53, 62, 68,
  69, 73–75, 80
RBE, 68, 73
RECIST, 147
Recurrent tumors, 238–241
Recursive partitioning analysis
  (RPA), 40, 46, 55,
  57–59, 61

Re-irradiation, 124, 126, 147
Renal and adrenal tumors,
        223–227
    adrenal gland metastases,
        226–227
    evidence, 224–227
    RCC, 223
Renal cell carcinoma (RCC), 5,
        139, 223–226
Reoxygenation, 6
Respiratory gating, 141
Retinopathy, 128
Review of systems, 48
Rhinorrhea, 44
Rib fracture, 146
Routine Quality Assurance
        Program, 28

S
Salvage, 58, 61
Salvage treatment, 45, 46, 73
Sarcoma, 139
Schwann cells, 41
Seizure, 40, 79
Seizure prophylaxis, 40
Sensorineural hearing loss, 48
Sensory changes, 48, 126, 146
Sex hormones, 41
Simpson grading system, 41
Simulation, 270
Simultaneous integrated boost
        (SIB), 173
Single-fraction photon radiation,
        3
Single metastasis, 55
Skull base paraganglioma, 69
Skull base tumor, 54
Smoking, 122
Soft tissue sarcoma
    dose prescription, 250–251
    evidence, 252–259
    follow-up, 251
    recommended imaging, 248
    simulation and treatment
        planning, 250

toxicities and management,
        251
treatment indications,
        248–250
Speech impairment, 80
Sphenoid, 45
Sphenopalatine ganglion, 45
Spinal cord, 132, 142
    compression and retreatment,
        104–105
    conventional EBRT, 101–102
    dose and technique, 97–100
    dose delivery, 93–96
    dose prescription, 93
    follow-up, 97
    late toxicity, 111–113
    pain flare, 109–110
    post-operative SBRT, 102–103
    primary tumors, 106–108
    simulation, 92–93
    toxicities and management,
        96–97
    treatment indications, 90
    treatment planning, 92–93
Spine, 126, 146
Spine metastases, 258
Spontaneous hemorrhage, 43, 72
Stereotactic photon therapy, 13
Staged SRS, 72
Standard fractionation, 5
Stent, 126
Stereotactic radiosurgery and
        stereotactic body
        radiotherapy (SRS/
        SBRT), 1, 43–47, 50,
        53–64, 67, 68, 70–72, 75,
        77–79, 122
    characteristics of, 18–21
    vs. conventional photon
        radiotherapy, 13
    cross-platform comparisons,
        17–25
    dose calculation algorithms,
        17
    hypofractionation techniques,
        5

IGRT solutions, 22–24
imaging techniques for, 13
immobilization devices, 12, 13
management of respiratory
        motion, 14
monotherapy, 216–218
patient safety, 25–30
patient setup, 12
plan classification, 16
plan optimization, 16
quality assurance, 25–30
treatment parameters, 14–16
treatment platforms, 17–25
Steroids, 40, 54, 56, 74, 79, 126,
        145, 146
STR, 47, 62
Stroke, 54
Superior mesenteric vein (SMV),
        173
Superior sulcus tumor, 138
Supportive care, 126, 146
Surgery, 47, 49, 58, 61–63, 65, 66,
        70, 71, 73, 76, 77
SVC syndrome, 138
Synchronous disease, 266

T
Temporal lobe, 79, 128
Testosterone, 48
Thalamotomy, 80
Thermoplastic mask, 12
Thoracentesis, 139
3-dimensional conformal
        radiation therapy
        (3D-CRT), 16

Thyroid/colorectal cancer, 139
Tinnitus, 41, 69
Tocopherol, 126, 146
Topical moisturizers, 126, 146
Transarterial chemoembolization
        (TACE), 163
Treatment planning system
        (TPS), 28
Tremor, 80
Trigeminal nerve, 44, 49, 50
Trigeminal neuralgia, 44, 54, 66,
        76–78
TSH, 42, 48

V
Vasculopathy, 126, 147
Vasomotor activity, 45
Venous sinus, 41
Ventralis intermedius, 80
Vertebral body compression
        fracture (VCF),
        108–109
Vertebral body metastasis, 94
Vertigo, 41, 69
Vestibular nerve, 41
Vestibular schwannoma, 41, 44,
        67, 68
Vision loss, 54
Visual field testing, 55
Vocal cord paralysis, 69

W
Weber tests, 48
WHO, 51, 61